### *Angels on the Night Shift*

"Excellent book. I read it in one evening. I had a fellow ER nurse borrow it as soon as I finished...Thank you for sharing this book with us."

—Ginger

"Fast-paced, fascinating, well-written, and absorbing...I thoroughly enjoyed this and will certainly be looking out for any other books written by this medical author."

—TheGardenWindow.blogspot.com

"I love your books! Always wondering who will burst through those doors next! Some of the stories are heartbreaking, some are encouraging, but all of them motivate me to become the best nurse possible. I can't wait for the next one!"

—Ruth

### *Angels and Heroes*

"Just wanted to say how much I am enjoying your books...as educational as well as inspirational respites from the day-to-day responsibilities of life...May God bless and keep you."

—Kim

"I am not one who likes to read, but when I started I could not put this book down...It made me realize that there are still good people on earth. I am a full-time police officer and a volunteer firefighter/EMS. I can't wait to pass this book on to others in my field."

—Gary

"What stories are held in this book—people who just go the whole way to be a help and sacrifice their lives! I am not much of a reader of nonfiction like this...but I fell in love with this book."

—GiveawayGal.blogspot.com

## Angels on Call

"Thank you for the amazingly awesome books you have written. As a Christian pursuing a career in medicine, I find them really inspiring. I had tears in my eyes many times, especially in *Angels on Call*. I love, love, love these books!"

—Alina

"As an assistant principal...I have reflected on my own life's work with adolescent students as I read each account...I am writing to share how very much I enjoyed your book, especially the inspiring scriptural references accompanying each story."

—Don

"The book was an inspiration during a difficult time in our lives...Your humility and humanity jumped out at me. I truly believe God works through us and that there are angels among us."

—Chuck

## Angels in the ER

"The most inspiring and relatable book I have read throughout my college career in nursing school...I often feel that my small contributions of extra time with patients or a simple smile have no impact on anyone's life. I was inspired by your book and appreciated the Bible verses throughout."

—Katie

"I am a busy working mother but managed to read the entire book in less than three days. The way you described the people and the situations was brilliant...You see things in a very special way and have made me see...thank you."

—Jamie

"Having spent ten years as a coordinator for our emergency department, I was very intrigued to read your stories...You have a very eloquent way of relating things that most people will never experience, but probably should...Your kindness, care, and compassion shine through."

—Alicia

# Ask the Family Doctor

### Robert D. Lesslie, MD
### &
### Robert Alexander, MD

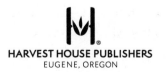

**HARVEST HOUSE PUBLISHERS**
EUGENE, OREGON

Cover design by Left Coast Design

Cover photos © file404 / shutterstock

When You Thought I Wasn't Looking © 2004. Mary Rita Schilke Korzan. Reprinted with permission of Andrews McMeel Publishing. All rights reserved.

Published in association with the Steve Laube Agency, LLC, 24 W. Camelback Rd. A 635, Phoenix, Arizona 85013.

This book is not intended to take the place of sound professional medical advice. Neither the author nor the publisher assumes any liability for possible adverse consequences as a result of the information contained herein.

## Ask the Family Doctor

Copyright © 2019 by Robert D. Lesslie, MD, and Robert Alexander, MD
Published by Harvest House Publishers
Eugene, Oregon 97408
www.harvesthousepublishers.com

ISBN 978-0-7369-7787-6 (pbk)
ISBN 978-0-7369-7788-3 (eBook)

Library of Congress Cataloging-in-Publication Data

Names: Lesslie, Robert D., 1951- author.
Title: Ask the family doctor : practical answers for medical situations every
     parent faces / Robert D. Lesslie, MD, Robert M. Alexander, MD.
Description: Eugene, Oregon : Harvest House Publishers, [2019]
Identifiers: LCCN 2019012132 (print) | LCCN 2019015497 (ebook) | ISBN
     9780736977883 (ebook) | ISBN 9780736977876 (paperback)
Subjects: LCSH: Medicine—Miscellanea. | Physicians—Miscellanea. | BISAC:
     RELIGION / Christian Life / Family.
Classification: LCC R706 (ebook) | LCC R706 .L4765 2019 (print) | DDC
     610—dc23
LC record available at https://lccn.loc.gov/2019012132

**Printed in the United States of America**

19  20  21  22  23  24  25  26  27  / BP-RD /  10  9  8  7  6  5  4  3  2  1

With thanksgiving for the blessings of our children
and for the parents they've become,
our efforts with this book are dedicated to

Lori and Rob, Amy and Dave, Robbie and Abby,
Jeff and Katie, Vance and Nicole,
Walt and Kim, and McAuley and Kara

Proverbs 4:23

Robert D. Lesslie, MD and Robert M. Alexander, MD

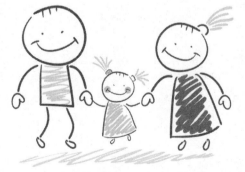

# Contents

# Help!

✚ *"Why don't children come with an instruction manual?"*

Parenting isn't just intimidating—it can be downright scary! As parents, we've willingly taken on the responsibility of providing for our children's nurture, safety, and well-being. And we've committed to doing that for a lot of years. Where *is* that instruction manual?

That's where we come in. Together we have more than 80 years of experience in answering those 2:00 a.m. phone calls and seeing thousands of children in the clinic or ER. In these pages we'll share a lot of what we've learned through those years—what to do, when to do it, and what to stay away from.

Between us we have seven children and seventeen grandchildren, so we've shared your midnight dilemmas and been where you are now.

Here's how we recommend using this book. You can read it straight through, flagging the questions that apply to you and your child right now, or you can check out the topical index and read about a problem you're currently facing. If you don't find what you're looking for, contact us at askthedox@yahoo.com, and we'll help you find an answer.

Robert M. Alexander, MD—Pediatrician

Robert D. Lesslie, MD—ER Physician

*"I think we've got this parenting gig NAILED."\**
*\*Said no parent ever."*

Lisa Maltby

# Love Languages

**✚ I don't understand my child,
and we're always knockin' heads! What can I do?**

*Simpatico*—"of similar mind or temperament." Sounds good, doesn't it? And wouldn't that make parenting a lot smoother? That's a worthy goal, to be of similar mind with your children, to understand where they're coming from and what makes them tick.

For some of us, that seems to come easy. But for most, it requires intentional effort. Fortunately, some people have thought through this challenge and offered help that's based on logic and outcomes. One such person is Gary Chapman, and he's given us a solid framework in his book *The 5 Love Languages*. It begins with suggesting you take a hard look at yourself to see what makes *you* tick. Once you've done that, you can focus on your child and build a long-lasting bridge of understanding and communication. The same goes for your spouse or any significant other. But we're going to focus on how to better understand your five- or fifteen-year-old.

> "Love is a choice you make every day."
>
> **GARY CHAPMAN**

We have limited space here, so we're just going to touch on Chapman's basic concepts. He outlines five types of "love languages"—ways we give and receive love. Each of us is unique, and while we have a primary love language, we might also have a blend with one or two others. These become manifest at an early age and remain with us throughout our lives. The key is to understand these five languages, identify which of them most closely applies to us, and then work to see which of them most closely applies to our children.

### Words of Affirmation

Right off the bat, we probably think of compliments when we see this one. And that would be correct. But there's much more to affirmation. Encouragement is an important part of it—"to inspire courage." And as Paul tells us in 1 Corinthians 13:4, "Love is kind." To show love, our words should be kind, gentle, and humble. How does your child respond to your words?

> "All of us blossom when we feel loved and wither when we do not feel loved."
>
> **GARY CHAPMAN**

### Quality Time

This one is tough. "Quality" means giving someone your undivided attention. Sitting in a movie theater together doesn't get it, nor does talking while both of you are texting away on your smartphones. Quality means focused attention and conversation, when the two of you are sharing feelings, thoughts, experiences, hopes, and dreams. When was the last time you and your "problem child" went somewhere and spent time one-on-one? And what happened?

### Receiving Gifts

Gifts can be visual symbols of love, and they don't have to be expensive. They just need to come from the heart. We're advocates of the adage "Don't give a child something they cry for," but this has nothing to do with that. It has everything to do with understanding that your child responds to symbols of your love, whether your gift is small but meaningful (maybe something he collects) or completely unexpected (like an outing for ice cream). It doesn't have to happen every day or every week, but if your child's love language is giving and receiving gifts, you have a lot of options and opportunities. When she gives you a gift, no matter the size or cost, stop what you're doing, think about it, and accept it as a demonstration of her love.

## Acts of Service

With children, this love language is most commonly expressed by the fulfillment of household chores. This delegation comes most effectively through requests and not orders. Remember that love is a choice and not a command. If your child's love language is acts of service, he'll show his love through *serving* you by completing his daily chores. You can do the same for him by helping with his chores or through small acts of service for him around the house. If children refuse to make their beds every morning, realize this might not be an act of rebellion or disrespect. It just might not be their love language. (Yet, that bed needs to be made, and that's another topic).

## Physical Touch

Obvious, isn't it? Most of us like and want to be touched, and for many, this is their primary love language. Small pats or hugs convey our love. Study your child's body language and response to your touch. If this is her love language, you'll be able to tell. And if that's the case, understand that excessive physical punishment can have long-term and disastrous consequences. If your daughter is upset and crying, the most important thing she needs is your presence and a hug.

That's it—our summary of Chapman's five love languages. If you and your child have the same love language—quality time, as an example—you're probably not "knockin' heads." And if you don't know your own language or that of your child, it might feel like you're just two ships passing in the night.

It doesn't have to be that way. If this idea of unique love languages strikes a chord, we wholeheartedly recommend that you get a copy of Chapman's book and study it. What you learn about your child and especially about yourself might be a surprise.

Simpatico. Work on it and get there.

*"Remember that your ultimate goal is for your children*
*to grow up secure in your love,*
*strong in their faith,*
*and with sound character."*

Gary Chapman

# Helicopter Moms and Aerial-Drone Dads

✚ *My sister says I'm a "helicopter mom,"*
*and I told her no way. Ahem. What's a helicopter mom?*

Groucho Marx is purported to have interviewed a mother of nine on his television show (circa 1950). When he learned how many children she had, he asked, "How in the world have you been able to manage so many kids without going crazy?"

"Well, it hasn't been easy. With our first child, my husband and I would rush him to the doctor with every sniffle, or scratch, or the slightest bruise. For a couple of months, we slept outside his door, listening for any change in his breathing or for any cough. He never left our sight. When number two came along, we did just about the same thing, except for sleeping outside her room. With number nine, it was different. One day when he swallowed a quarter, we just took it out of his allowance."

That story is a good example of the evolution of a "helicopter mom"—constantly hovering over her child—to a more relaxed yet competent parent. The term has been around for a couple of decades, but it's recently gained more attention. That might be because of its increasing incidence and the mounting evidence that it does more harm than good to a child.

Helicopter parenting refers to a style of being overly focused on our children, especially their perceived needs and specifically on their successes and failures. "Overparenting" is a way of describing it, referring to overprotecting and overcontrolling. The logical extension is to become a "Black Hawk parent," referring to the military assault type of helicopter. This would mean employing all opportunities and avenues to secure the most favorable outcome possible for your child regardless of the scorched earth left behind.

Another term for an overparenting parent is "lawn mower." This is the mother or father who will mow down any obstacle, problem, frustration, or inconvenience that might stand in the way of their child and his or her success. "Cosseting" is a gentler term, implying that the parent wraps a child in cotton wool to protect them, but the goals and outcomes are the same. We like the term "smother" because it's descriptive and kind of cute.

> "We're raising children who have little tolerance for disappointment."
>
> **AUTHOR UNKNOWN**

All these terms can be applied to the parent of a child of almost any age. Toddlers can be overparented, as well as middle-schoolers and teenagers. Now that this issue is being discussed more openly, there is growing concern that overparenting extends to our children's college years and beyond.

Why do parents hover? Why do we feel compelled to overparent and overprotect? Most of the many reasons start in a good place and grow into something unhealthy. We worry about our child not succeeding—not making good grades in school, not excelling in sports or any other extracurricular activity, not getting into the right school or college, not getting the right job. We worry about her being disappointed and fear she might—heaven help us—fail in some endeavor. Some of us might have felt unloved or neglected when we were growing up, and we don't want our child to feel that way. And sometimes we see other parents overparenting, and we feel pressured and compelled to do the same. What starts as good intentions can quickly turn into unhealthy actions.

### ✦ What's unhealthy about wanting to protect my child?

Nothing—until it becomes obsessive. Being involved with our

children gives them a sense of self-worth, love, and acceptance, but too much involvement deprives them of the chance to sort things out on their own. Instead of self-worth and self-confidence, we instill feelings of doubt and indecision. And when we don't allow them to fail, we deny them the chance to learn new skills that will help them handle challenges and failures—both of which they will face repeatedly throughout their lives. In addition to fostering a decreased self-confidence and self-esteem, overparenting prevents our children from developing constructive coping skills—handling the bumps in the road they will face every day. And recent evidence suggests that children who are overparented will have more anxiety and an increased risk for depression. On top of all that, the presence in the home of a helicopter mom or aerial-drone dad produces stress for all family members and increases the potential for marital discord.

> "A child needs both to be hugged and unhugged. The hug lets her know she is valuable. The unhug lets her know that she is viable. If you're always shoving your child away, they will cling to you for love. If you're always holding them closer, they will cling to you for fear."
>
> **POLLY BERRIEN BERENDS**

### ✦ Maybe my sister's right. Maybe I am a helicopter mom. I don't think I'm a Black Hawk yet, but how can I know?

Being appropriately involved with your children and protecting them when needed and not slipping down the slope of excessive sheltering is a delicate balance. Malinda Carlson, in her article "10 Warning Signs That You Might Be a Helicopter Parent (and How to Stop)," gives us some informative and challenging guidance. She says you might be a helicopter parent if you recognize some of these ten signs:

1. You only let your child play on playgrounds with shredded rubber mulch.

2. The first thing you did when your fourth grader came

home crying from school because her best friend Jill called her a name is to call Jill's mom to sort things out yourself.

3. You have found yourself up at 11 p.m. rewriting your child's English essay because you know that she could have done a better job if she hadn't been so tired.

4. Your eight-year-old still has training wheels on his bike. Not that you let him ride it that often. The sidewalks are dangerous, and they go too fast for you to keep up!

5. You have a bad back from stooping down and following your toddler's every step.

6. You get heart palpitations at the thought of letting your child go on a field trip with their class.

7. Having them help out by preparing dinner or cleaning the house has never crossed your mind. Knives are sharp and the cleaning fluids are too dangerous!

8. As a Christmas gift you gave your daycare a webcam so you could watch the daily happenings while you're at work.

9. You and your son have a meeting with the teacher, and when she asks him a question you answer it for him.

10. Your child didn't get accepted to his preferred major at college, so you call the chair of the department to negotiate for an exception.[1]

We don't have to be guilty of all of these to be a helicopter mom or an aerial-drone dad, but you get the picture. Now what do we do about it?

The first thing is to step back to see if this describes how you parent. When your child is playing soccer, football, or T-ball, are you behind the fence or on the field? If you're on the field and in the coach's or ref's ear, you might be "cosseting"—or worse. Make a list of what you do that might qualify as overparenting. Consider getting some help from that sister of yours, a teacher, or your spouse. Maybe you're helping your child complete a puzzle when she becomes frustrated. Back off and give her more time. Go down your list and eliminate a few things at a time. Allow your child to fail, and then teach him he doesn't have to be perfect. Children need to work at things, but they don't have to be perfect and always finish in first place.

Perhaps the hardest thing is to let them fight their own battles. Yes, we need to guard our children from obviously dangerous encounters. However, letting them deal with the everyday skirmishes and struggles of this life will equip them with the skills they'll need when you're no longer in the next room.

It comes down to what we want to accomplish with our parenting. Do we want our children to be "safe," protected from every possible difficulty? Or do we want them to be strong, self-assured, and grounded?

We hope even a lawn-mower dad can answer that one.

> *"There's a lot of ugly things in this world, son.*
> *I wish I could keep 'em all away from you.*
> *That's never possible."*
>
> Atticus Finch, *To Kill a Mockingbird*

# 3

# Vaccinations

➕ *I've always been fine with having my children vaccinated.*
*But lately I've been looking at the internet, and...well,*
*I'm just not sure. I don't know if it's safe.*

We're not sure what you've been reading, but we can imagine. Vaccination naysayers have been around for as long as we've had vaccinations, and we've had them for 200 years. They started with the Englishman Edward Jenner and his discovery of using the cowpox virus to prevent smallpox. In the eighteenth century, smallpox killed more than 400,000 Europeans *yearly* and caused blindness, deafness, and disfigurement in hundreds of thousands more. It was highly lethal, killing more than 80 percent of the children who were infected.

Despite Jenner's work and the promise of preventing this infection, though, he was persecuted by a fervent group of "vaccine hesitant" individuals. Thankfully, smallpox is gone, but not because we figured out how to kill the virus. Rather, we developed a vaccine that boxed it into a corner and then finally into a couple of test tubes hidden away somewhere.

The effectiveness of the smallpox vaccine, as well as that of many other vaccines currently in use, has fostered a lot of the opposition to the idea of vaccination in general. People fall victim to the "out of sight, out of mind" mentality. They no longer see the infections that routinely swept across this country, such as polio and measles. These are still serious problems in other areas of the world, but most of us in the United States have no experience with them. As an example, prior to an effective vaccine, measles killed 500 Americans each year and was the reason for 48,000 hospitalizations and 1,000 cases of permanent brain damage annually. Even today, 146,000 people will die from measles this year worldwide. We've lost sight of how dangerous this virus is.

And speaking of measles, an outbreak in the Pacific Northwest, centered in Washington, continues as we write this chapter. To date, more than 50 cases of measles have been documented, most in unvaccinated individuals. This virus is highly contagious, and it's thought that the transmission rate is near 100 percent when an unvaccinated person comes in contact with the virus. How does this kind of outbreak happen? Well, it seems that a lot of parents don't think it's important to have their children (or themselves) immunized. They've joined the same "vaccine hesitant" camp Edward Jenner faced. When enough people join that camp, our "herd immunity" is no longer effective. Let's consider what we mean by herd immunity.

Suppose we have 100 head of cattle (our herd). If enough of them are vaccinated or are immune to a specific infectious disease—say, measles—the disease might affect one or two of the animals but won't spread among those who are immune. The infected cows get over it (or die), and the measles fritter away. A critical number of immune cows are needed to cause that frittering, and it seems to be in the neighborhood of 90 percent. Less than that, and the herd is not immune and the infection spreads. In many parts of the country, vaccination rates exceed 97 percent, conferring significant herd immunity. In the area where we're seeing this outbreak, estimates of vaccination against the measles virus is less than 40 percent—an outbreak waiting to happen, and it did.

What might be causing this parental vaccine hesitancy? We believe it's the dissemination of misleading or inaccurate information. In fact, if the internet could be vaccinated against bogus medical advice, we'd all be better off.

So what is the truth here? What's factual and what's not? We state categorically that childhood vaccinations are effective and lifesaving. That's been proven over and over. But as we noted, this very effectiveness is what allows some of us to lose sight of the dangers of whooping cough, polio, diphtheria, pneumonia, meningitis, and other previously common infections. We also affirm that these vaccines are safe. Some risks are involved, and those need to be considered, but what are they? Let's start with how they are *not* a risk.

*Do vaccinations cause autism?* There is *no* evidence to link vaccinations—specifically the MMR—with autism. None. And there's no evidence that the mercury-containing preservative thimerosal is connected with autism. The confusion arose because some people believed that thimerosal acted like another, more toxic form of mercury does. But thimerosal has been proven safe. (Cautious parents should be aware, however, that some vaccines free of this preservative are available.)

*Do vaccinations cause type 1 diabetes or Bell's palsy?* Contrary to what you might find on the internet, there is also no evidence that the MMR, diphtheria-tetanus, or pertussis vaccines are causally related to the onset of type 1 diabetes. Likewise, no evidence exists that links the flu vaccine to the development of Bell's palsy.

*Are vaccinations administered too close together?* A more recent parental concern relates to the safety of established immunization schedules. The concern is that too many vaccines are given over too short a period of time and that a child's immune system can be overwhelmed. That concern has only grown with the addition of other effective vaccines, such as those for hepatitis, the rotavirus, meningitis, and HPV. Most of the population views these additional vaccines as a huge victory for our public health.

However, some nonmedical *and* medical people believe in administering these vaccinations over a longer period of time. Yet the reality is that the current schedule is designed to protect children against diseases *when they are the most susceptible.* If this period of susceptibility is drawn out, we'll see more infections. And as far as "overwhelming" our immune systems, there is no evidence to suggest that possibility. In fact, a group of researchers suggest that the newborn's immune system could safely respond to up to 10,000 vaccines at a time.[1] (We'd hate to be in that clinic!)

Now that we've addressed some common misperceptions about vaccinations, let's consider what we know to be actual but small or rare risks.

*Increased incidence of febrile seizures.* In our chapter on febrile seizures (chapter 7), we note an increased incidence of these seizures after the MMR vaccine. This increased risk is small, however, and we note that most experts recommend giving the next dose of MMR regardless of a previous febrile seizure.

*Serious allergic reactions.* Serious allergic reactions (anaphylaxis) are possible with many of these vaccines, including the tetanus, chicken pox, MMR, hepatitis B, and flu vaccines. The risk is small, only 0.65 cases per 1 million doses. Many components of a vaccine can be the culprit for an allergic reaction, including the antigen itself, preservatives, egg proteins, yeast, gelatin, and latex. It's rare, but it can happen.

Local reactions commonly occur in up to 50 percent of those being vaccinated. They depend on the specific vaccine and include localized redness, pain, swelling, and a mild fever. These reactions usually go away on their own in a couple of days without any treatment.

*Joint pain.* There is weak evidence to suggest that the MMR vaccine can cause joint pain in women and children, but if it happens, it doesn't last long.

We believe it's most important for parents to consider these two key points:

1. Vaccine-preventable diseases are dangerous, and they can kill.

2. Vaccinations are safe and effective.

Benjamin Franklin's haunting words are timely and still ring true more than 250 years later:

> In 1736 I lost one of my sons, a fine boy of four years old, by the small-pox, taken in the common way. I long regretted bitterly, and still regret that I had not given it to him by inoculation.

If you're interested in more information, forget the internet unless you're consulting one of these sites:

- www.CDC.gov/vaccines—Search the site for vaccine information statements or a list of precautions for commonly used vaccines.
- Vaccinate Your Family—www.ecbt.org
- Immunization Action Coalition—www.immunize.org
- Vaccinate Your Baby—www.vaccinateyourbaby.com
- Voices for Vaccines—www.voicesforvaccines.org
- Children's Hospital of Philadelphia Vaccine Education Center—https://www.chop.edu/centers-programs/vaccine-education-center
- AAP.org—This is the American Academy of Pediatrics website.

Jonathan Swift, the author of *Gulliver's Travels*, didn't know about the internet, but he understood human nature:

> *"Falsehood flies, and the truth comes limping after it;*
> *so that when men come to be undeceived, it is too late;*
> *the jest is over, and the tale has had its effect."*

# 4

# Bullying

*✤ We think our eight-year-old boy is being bullied at school. His grades are slipping, and he doesn't want to ride the bus anymore. He won't talk about it. What should we do?*

If you haven't read—or seen the film version of—*How Green Was My Valley*, a novel by Richard Llewellyn, you need to add it to your bucket list. In the movie, actor Roddy McDowall plays the young son of a Welsh coal miner who's being bullied at his new school. He's coming home with black eyes, bruises, and a wounded ego. His older brothers—grown men and coal miners themselves—procure the services of a wiry, experienced prizefighter who teaches their brother the art of boxing. In short order, the bullies have been leveled and all is well. It's a feel-good moment, but the reality of bullying and its outcomes are not always so straightforward. Here's a more typical example.

> Wes Wood and his family recently moved to Rock Hill, where Wes's father is a senior vice president at one of the local banks. Wes is 12 years old, tall and slender, and not very athletic. Since the age of eight, he's had a tic—squeezing his eyes closed, pursing his lips, and jerking his head to the left. It had improved over the past year or so with the help of their pediatrician and a counselor; the episodes had become much less frequent and could be traced to some precipitating stressful event. But his parents anticipated the stress of a new city and a new school, so they worked with Wes to identify and deal with any feelings of anxiety he might experience.

That seemed to be working...for a while. He was always a good student—honor roll in all of his previous classes—and things started out the same way in Rock Hill. But then two months into the school year, his grades began to slip and his tic returned. His parents had found a good pediatrician in Rock Hill, and the doctor quickly identified the problem when Wes was forthcoming about the bullying he was experiencing in school. Several boys picked on him because of his tic and made fun of his skinniness. At first this took the form of verbal taunts, but recently the boys had begun to physically abuse him. They employed painful pinches, leaving bruises in areas under clothing where they wouldn't be obvious to a casual observer.

The mother of one of his classmates called Wes's parents and identified the perpetrators after her own son expressed concern about what was happening. They asked for a meeting with the school principal and the three boys. There, Wes's parents were surprised to learn that the three offenders were all honor students. They were also clean cut and polite, and the father of one of them worked at Wes's father's bank. They admitted to bullying Wes. Now what?

Bullying has been the topic of a lot of conversations recently. It's nothing new, but we're beginning to understand more about it and the seriousness of its consequences. It can take many forms, but at its heart, bullying is a type of aggression where one or more children repeatedly and intentionally harass or physically harm someone who is perceived to be weak and unable to defend himself. The important points here are *repetition* over time and the *unequal power relationship*. Those will be the common factors in any form of bullying. The victim will perceive herself as being weaker than the bully and unable to put up a defense.

It's not just physical abuse. Bullying includes being threatened, verbally abused (name-calling), socially isolated or the subject of rumors, and, increasingly, targeted in the growing arena of social media.

This is way too common, with estimates that at any one point in time, as many as 10 percent of children are being regularly bullied. Just as troubling is that up to as many as 90 percent of adolescents will face physical or psychological bullying before leaving high school. Obtaining accurate numbers is difficult for several reasons. Frequently, bullying goes unreported, with as many as half of those being bullied not telling anyone—especially boys, older children, and those who are bullied infrequently.

As a general rule, boys are about 50 percent more frequently involved in bullying than girls, and boys are more frequently the target of *physical* abuse. Girls are more often the targets or perpetrators of nonphysical bullying, such as the spreading of rumors, gossip, and smear campaigns using their social media outlets, which is just as painful. Most of this bullying happens during the second through ninth grades, with the highest incidence occurring at age seven.

> "I think parenting these days is definitely different from when a lot of people grew up...Bullying was one-on-one and face-to-face. Now it's all over the internet."
>
> **NELLY**

### ✤ What does a bully look and act like?

As we see in Wes's case, there isn't a stereotype for a bully. They come in all shapes and sizes. We do know that many are aggressive toward their teachers, parents, siblings, and classmates and are quicker to resort to physical and violent means to exert their dominance over others and to control their sphere of influence. If they're male, they're more likely to be bigger and stronger than most of their classmates—especially those they seek to bully.

But contrary to what we might think, they usually don't bully from a sense of insecurity or a lack of self-esteem. Wes's bullies were school leaders, accomplished in the classroom and on the athletic field. What they did have in common with just about every bully was the desire and need for power and domination. Girls do the same thing, but as we've noted, usually without the physical component. As we might expect, children who are physically aggressive tend to lack both social skills *and* empathy, while those who use social means of bullying tend to lack empathy but are socially skilled. The more intelligent, older, and socially sophisticated bullies are more likely to get away with aggressive behavior. They learn how to avoid detection.

### ✤ What about the victims? What do they look like?

As you might expect, bullied kids seem to be more passive and insecure than their peers. They tend to be smaller, weaker, more sensitive, and quiet. They are frequently loners, whether by nature or social circumstance. The important thing to remember is that there is no typical victim just as there is no typical bully. Many victims seem to be successful and self-assured students, and many bullies are class leaders, charming, and well versed in the social graces.

Bullying can occur anywhere, but it's most frequent in our schools— when and where there is the least adult supervision. The playground is a common site. In primary schools, victims are frequently bullied during breaks, lunchtime, or recess. In secondary grades, this happens in hallways, classrooms, and bathrooms. Bathrooms are problematic, causing many victims to avoid school restrooms because of their fear of being assaulted. And, again, this is a location where there is little if any adult supervision.

### ✤ What are the consequences of bullying if it only scares kids?

Scaring them is enough, isn't it? Some children spend their entire school experience living in fear and anxiety. This can lead to poor self-esteem, social isolation, poor academic performance, depression, and, in the extreme, suicide and other violent actions. We've read about increasing episodes of violent retaliation, which includes suicide, prompted by chronic anxiety and feelings of powerlessness.

The consequences of bullying are serious, and they don't affect just the victim. Those who bully have ongoing social problems that extend into young adulthood and beyond. Some estimates indicate that as many as two-thirds of boys who bully will have at least one criminal conviction by the time they're 24 years old, and one-third will have three or more convictions by that age. While it's important not to stereotype a bully (or a victim), the evidence clearly indicates the need to identify any antisocial or aggressive behavior early and deal with it.

So how do we identify this problem? Children will tell their parents about being bullied more often than their teachers will observe or volunteer this information. This could be caused by their having too many students to properly supervise or, as some studies indicate, being inadequately prepared to handle bullying. With that in mind, we need to be open about this and discuss it with our kids when we have any concerns. Signs of being bullied include difficulty sleeping, vague abdominal pain, new onset or recurrence of bed-wetting, headaches, moodiness, and more visits to the school nurse. If your child has a chronic medical condition or behavior problem (Wes's tics), he or she can become a target for bullying, so pay special attention in these circumstances.

Here are some questions to ask your child if you suspect he is being bullied:

- Are you being picked on or teased at school?
- What do other children pick on you about?
- How long has this been going on?
- Have you told your teacher?
- Do you feel safe at recess, or do you tend to stay by yourself?
- Are any of your friends or classmates being bullied?

As parents, we need to be aware. We should ask ourselves:

- Do I have any concern that my child is having difficulties with classmates at school? Has the thought of her being bullied ever crossed my mind?

- Has a teacher ever mentioned that my kid tends to isolate herself, especially during recess?
- Does my child make frequent visits to the school nurse?
- Have I missed subtle comments that might indicate bullying?

### ✚ I've talked with my child, and I'm convinced he's being bullied at school. Now what?

It's time to act, and that means talking with his teachers. Without an active adult intervention, this problem won't go away. If a teacher isn't aware of what's going on or appears to downplay the problem, go to the principal. Fortunately, there is a heightened awareness of this issue in our schools, and most teachers and school officials are sensitive to its seriousness. Many legal cases across the country have even affirmed the following "rights for school victims":

- to be protected against foreseeable criminal activity
- to be protected against student crime or violence that can be prevented by adequate supervision
- to be protected from dangerous individuals negligently placed in schools
- to be protected against identifiable dangerous students[1]

We expect adults to be protected from this kind of behavior. Don't we want our children to be protected too? It can be done. A comprehensive school-wide anti-bullying campaign and strategy can successfully lower the incidence of bullying and aggressive behavior, regardless of the social or ethnic makeup of the school. It just takes knowledge, commitment, and consistent action.

In addition to encouraging their children to report *every* episode of bullying to an adult, parents can do some other things to help kids deal with this problem. For instance, we know victims of bullying frequently project a sense of weakness, insecurity, and passivity, and we can help them with that.

First, we can let them know that this demeanor can invite more bullying. Standing tall, speaking in a strong, clear voice, and making direct eye contact will all help. Employing a "walk, talk, squawk" response might help as well: *Walk* away from the bully, not run. *Talk* directly to the bully, making direct eye contact and using a confident voice and words (that's going to take some time to master and can be taught through role-playing at home), and then *squawk*—tell a teacher or another adult what happened. Again, your child needs to be encouraged to do this. Kids need to understand that adults are available to protect them.

Second, if our children's self-esteem is being damaged, we need to address that as well. Helping them identify something they can be successful doing is a good start. This may be a sport, participation in a club at school, or some opportunity involving music. Not only will this help them build self-confidence; it will also broaden their social circles in a positive way.

If we think our child is a bully or we've been confronted by teachers or other adults saying that he's demonstrating abusive behavior toward other children, the worst thing we can do is become defensive. We need to investigate this completely and become involved. If we leave his bullying unaddressed, we will fail to provide him with the chance to constructively deal with a problem that will shadow him for life.

Bullying is a serious problem for everyone involved. This should always be a zero-tolerance issue wherever it's occurring. It needs to be dealt with head-on, and if we do that, we can help our children—victims and bullies alike.

If you want more information, check out the app the Substance Abuse and Mental Health Services Administration (SAMHSA) has for downloading at www.store.samhsa.gov. Then search "bullying."

*"It is easier to build strong children than to repair broken men."*

Frederick Douglass

# 5

# When to Go to the ER

✚ *When should I take my child to the ER?*
*I don't want to be an alarmist, but I don't want to miss*
*something important either.*

That's a great question, and one the ER doctor here (Dr. Lesslie) wishes more people asked. Knowing when life and limb are threatened and when they aren't comes down to common sense and understanding. We understand the panic when your child is experiencing a sudden and unexpected problem or has fallen with blood seemingly everywhere. Our advice is to always err on the side of caution, which in this instance means safety. Here are some scenarios that warrant an evaluation in the ER of a hospital:

- Anything that affects the airway. This could be sudden choking (think *foreign body*), wheezing, croup in an infant, duskiness of the skin (from lack of oxygen), or chest wall retractions. In short, be aware of anything that makes you worry about your child getting enough air.
- cuts/lacerations that spurt or won't stop bleeding
- A new seizure (we address febrile seizures in chapter 7).
- confusion
- an unstable gait
- loss of consciousness
- Ingestion of OTC (over-the-counter) or prescription medication (call your Poison Control Center immediately).

- new and severe abdominal pain
- new and severe headache
- vomiting that won't stop for 10 to 12 hours or evidence that your child is becoming dehydrated
- evidence of shock—rapid heart rate, skin duskiness, and cool/damp skin

This is a good time to talk about a fast heartbeat. This can be a red flag for the presence of several bad things, so we need to know what we're looking for. If the child is agitated and crying, that's going to raise his heart rate, and the number you get probably won't be of much help. Here are the ranges:

  - 0 to 3 months—up to 165 beats/minute

  - 3 to 6 months—160

  - 6 to 12 months—150

  - 1 to 2 years—135

  - 2 to 3 years—130

  - 3 to 6 years—120

  - 6 years and older—100 to 110

Take your child's pulse when he or she is well, calm, and rested. You can do this over the carotid artery (neck) or at the wrist. It's best to count for a full minute, but at the very least, allow 30 seconds. (Don't forget to multiply by two.) Along with a temperature reading, this is a helpful vital sign to provide your pediatrician, especially during one of those 2:00 a.m. emergency phone calls.

- fever "of concern"

Not every fever is cause for alarm, but here are the temperatures that should prompt a call or visit to your pediatrician, or if she's not available, a trip to the ER:

- Birth to 3 months—100.4 or greater (By the way, all temperatures in this book are expressed in Fahrenheit degrees.)
- 3 to 36 months—102.2 or greater
- Older children—103.1 or greater

- a fever combined with a severely angulated fracture or a fracture that pokes through the skin
- a fever accompanied by a widespread rash

Use common sense, but if you have any concern for your child's safety, get some help. Quickly.

Perhaps we can gain more perspective into the appropriate use of the ER by considering when *not* to go. You might think this would be obvious to everyone, but no, that's not the case. Here are some real cases and complaints that just might prove that point:

- A three-year-old has pinworms, and Mom wants the entire family checked for them—at 2:00 a.m.
- An eight-year-old has ringworm and is brought to the ER for help—in the middle of the night.
- Dad presents with his teenage daughter at midnight. She needs a school sports physical for cheerleader tryouts—the next day.
- Mom brings her three children in "to be checked" after a minor fender bender. They weren't involved in the wreck, but they watched it happen, and she's concerned that they're upset.
- There's a lice outbreak in one of the local schools, and a mother brings in her three children and two nephews just to be sure they don't have them.
- A 13-year-old smoked marijuana at a friend's house and now feels "funny."

- As she pats her two-year-old on the head, a mom says, "I can't find my wedding ring, so I want you to x-ray my boy. He has a habit of putting things in his mouth."

- A parent says, "My ten-year-old has had a sore throat for a couple of hours, and I didn't want to bother our family doctor." It's 2:00 a.m.

- A new mother says, "I just noticed my baby has blue eyes, and my boyfriend's eyes are brown. I want a DNA test."

- A parent explains, "Doctor, I saw a medical special about a rare disease on TV last night, and I think my boy has all the symptoms. My neighbor thinks so too. She even thinks I've got it." Or even worse, a mom comes in saying, "Doc, I watched a commercial this afternoon about one of the drugs I'm taking. They said you shouldn't take it if you're pregnant, but I did. I've been on a medicine similar to it for a long time and took it while I was pregnant, and I need to have my son checked out." She then points to her 18-year-old, seated beside her on the stretcher. Yes, it happened...and there's more.

> "Each generation has been an education for us in different ways. The first child with a bloody nose was rushed to the ER. The fifth child with a bloody nose was told to go to the yard immediately and stop bleeding on the carpet."
>
> **ART LINKLETTER**

- "I need an ultrasound to find out if my baby is a boy or a girl."

- "Our dog has mange, and we all [two adults and four children] need to be checked."

- "I think my child has a fever, but our thermometer's broken." (Meanwhile, the four-year-old is just finishing his fifth lap around the ER.)

- A request for a second opinion for a ten-year-old regarding the necessity of an elective surgical procedure that was recommended six months ago by a doctor two states away.

- A request for a school note for a second grader because the parent was hung over from the previous weekend and couldn't get him to school for two days.

- A parent was worried about a 16-year-old's 30-pound weight gain over the past two months. (Oops…was that a candy bar that fell out of her jacket pocket? Wait, there's another one.)

- Super Bowl Sunday and, unfortunately, another actual case. When the father of three young children was asked why he brought them to the ER, his response was, "I guess to get them checked out, but, really, you guys get better TV reception in the waiting room than I do at my house."

So when should you take your child to the ER? Be guided by some knowledge—and a little common sense.

*"Common sense is like deodorant. The ones who need it most don't use it."*

Author Unknown

# 6

# Fever

*✚ Our two-year-old has a fever of 102,*
*and my aunt told us to put him in a bath of ice water.*
*How long should we leave him in there?*

What?

Our answer? Make sure your aunt reads this chapter. We're going to provide you with a good understanding of "fever" and, we hope, release you (and your aunt!) from a pervasive problem called "fever phobia." Let's start with the basics.

Our body temperatures are controlled by a specific location in our brains—the hypothalamus. Here resides the "thermoregulatory center," which balances heat production and heat loss. This is important to keep in mind because it's the site of action for the drugs we use to lower our temperature. This center maintains our body temperatures in a normal range despite environmental factors such as cold and heat. We have a "set point" for this that we're able to adjust using increased metabolic activity (in a cold environment) and sweating (in a hot environment). When we have a fever, it's this "set point" that gets messed up, usually because of some kind of infection. Our brains reset to what they think our new normal temperature should be.

If asked what's a normal temperature, most of us would answer 98.6 degrees. And we would be right—probably. This number comes from several studies done in the nineteenth century. More recent information indicates that normal body temperatures vary with age, level of activity, time of day, and even with the phase of a woman's menstrual cycle. It seems that an upper limit of normal would be 98.9 degrees in the morning and 99.9 overall. We know that infants and young children have higher "normal" temperatures than older children and adults. For instance, in the newborn period (age 0 to 28 days), the average normal temperature is about 99.5 degrees, with an upper limit of 100.4. So technically in this age group, 100.0 is *not* a fever. This normal range increases a little as a child gets older, but only a little. As mentioned before, normal temperature varies during the day, with our lowest occurring in the morning. Temperatures peak in the late afternoon or evening, and the variation can be as much as 1.8 degrees. Keep this in mind when you're monitoring your child's temperature.

### ✛ What's the best way to check my child's temperature? I see all kinds of methods on the internet.

Those of us who have or have had children under five know taking their temperature can be a challenge. The easiest method is a tympanic membrane (TM) thermometer inserted in the ear or maybe one of the forehead devices placed on the skin. But that would be the wrong answer to the question "What's the best way?" Though they're easy and nonthreatening, they're also too inaccurate to be of real help. Save your money.

Aside from those options, we have the choice of a rectal, oral, or axillary (armpit) temperature. The gold standard is the rectal route up until age five. After that, an oral temperature is the first choice (if the child will cooperate), followed by an axillary temperature. Let's consider these methods.

A rectal temperature is the basis for most medical studies and is the most accurate measurement of our core temperature. If we're going to base significant medical decisions on our temperature measurement, we want it to be as accurate as possible. Those decisions can lead to extensive workups, including X-rays, lab studies, and even spinal taps.

Oral thermometers are preferred by a child who is old enough to cooperate, but the readings can be affected by the recent ingestion of hot or cold liquids. Make sure you wait at least 15 minutes after your child has had something to drink or eat before taking a temperature. Also, the child needs to keep the thermometer in a closed mouth during the entire process. Mouth breathing will yield an inaccurate reading. As beginning physicians, we were taught that an oral temperature is typically 1 degree cooler than a rectal measurement, and that still seems to be the rule.

An axillary measurement can be used (with your oral thermometer—not rectal), but the reading will be consistently lower than a rectal reading. This difference varies too much to come up with an agreed-upon number, but it may be as much as 2 degrees cooler. This temperature gives us some information, but it's limited. If it's critical to know the core temperature of a child, the rectal temperature is still the best.

Now that we've measured our child's temperature, what constitutes a fever? Most experts agree that a fever is an abnormal elevation of temperature that results from our brain (remember the hypothalamus) responding to several changes in our body, the most common a viral or bacterial infection. This abnormal elevation depends on the age of your child, how the temperature was measured, and what might be causing the elevation.

In most instances, the height of a temperature is less important than the appearance of the child and the presence of worrisome symptoms such as irritability, a stiff neck, or lethargy. It's important to know what we consider to be fevers of concern. Temperatures in this area will prompt a more extensive examination and search for a specific cause. These ranges assume that your child has been previously healthy.

- 0 to 3 months of age—a *rectal* temperature equal to or greater than 100.4 degrees

- 3 months to 6 months of age—a *rectal* temperature equal to or greater than 102.2 degrees

- older children—an *oral* temperature equal to or greater than 103.1 degrees

What's going on here? We mentioned our brain's temperature set point. When inflammatory chemicals are released by the actions of viruses, bacteria, and even our own white blood cells, they travel to our brains and reset our set point to a higher level. Our body responds by doing what it's supposed to do—raise our temperature to the new set point. Our brain sends signals to increase metabolism (hence the shivering we experience with a fever) and increase muscle tone and activity. This goes on until we reach the new mark. The upper limit seems to be 107.6 degrees. That's a scary number. This can happen with heatstroke, but it's usually limited to 106.0 degrees without something external going on. Still, pretty scary.

### ✚ I've always been told that our brains fry at a temperature of 105! That's why we need to treat every fever our child has, right?

Nope, and not necessarily. Fever does *not* cause brain damage even in the extreme. And we're going to consider when and if a fever needs to be treated at all.

Some researchers think fever can be our friend. First, some evidence indicates that an elevated temperature can slow the growth and multiplication of certain bacteria and viruses. And because fever is a normal response to those inflammatory chemicals we mentioned, it might have additional roles in fighting infection, such as improving our immune response. These possible benefits are minimal, however, and in some circumstances fever does more harm than good. It makes us uncomfortable and irritable. It increases our metabolic rate (again, shivering is an example), thus placing increased demands on our heart and lungs. For previously healthy children, this is not a significant factor, but it's significant in the child with a heart condition or with a condition like asthma.

Because fever is a sign of an underlying disease process, we need to determine its cause. Frequently, it's a simple viral infection, but it could be something more serious, such as a bacterial infection.

### ✚ I've heard that if my child's fever goes down with acetaminophen, it's most likely a viral infection because this won't happen with a bacterial problem.

We've heard that, too, and it's dead wrong. A child's response to acetaminophen or ibuprofen won't help distinguish between a viral or bacterial infection. We wish it did. That would make all our lives simpler. That's one important point we need to be aware of regarding our approach to fever. Here are some others, a few of which we've already mentioned:

- Fever is not a disease or illness; it's a normal bodily response.

- There is no evidence that fever—no matter its height—makes an illness worse.

- Most fevers in previously healthy children are self-limited—they will resolve on their own.

- Fever does not cause brain damage.

- The first things to do to reduce a child's elevated temperature are to provide extra fluids and reduce physical activity (children will usually become less active on their own).

- If a child is uncomfortable because of the fever, that's an indication it needs to be treated.

- If your child has a fever and you're treating it, don't wake them up to give them their fever medicine.

- Pay attention to other medications your child is taking, such as cough and cold preparations. Many of these contain acetaminophen or ibuprofen and can lead to an accidental overdose if combined with more acetaminophen or ibuprofen to bring down a fever.

- Fever medications are given according to *weight*, not age. This is important because dosing by age can lead to under- or overdosing. Ask your physician for a 5 or 10 cc syringe to help you with accurate dosing. The ones provided with OTC medications are frequently inaccurate.

Fever medications act by restoring the thermoregulatory set point we talked about at the beginning of this chapter. We have a couple of these medicines, with acetaminophen and ibuprofen the most commonly used. Aspirin falls into this category but shouldn't be used because of its association with Reye's syndrome in children and teenagers (brain swelling, vomiting, confusion, seizures, liver failure—something none of us want). Make sure you check the contents of any of your children's OTC medications in your medicine cabinet. Throw out anything with aspirin in it.

Before you decide to start a child on one of these medicines, keep in mind that routinely treating every fever in an otherwise healthy and normal child is not always indicated. Fever isn't a disease. There's no evidence that reducing fever will improve the duration or severity of the underlying cause. In addition, use of these medicines can lead to drug toxicity and may delay the identification of a serious infection.

However, reducing your child's fever *can* improve their discomfort and might reduce the risk of dehydration through less water loss from sweating. It's a case-by-case decision, but because most of these decisions are made by parents without the consultation of their family doctor, be sure you know as much about these medications as you can.

Most pediatricians recommend acetaminophen as their first choice for treating fever. It has a long track record for safety (when dosed correctly), and it's effective in lowering an elevated temperature. Ibuprofen is effective as well—maybe slightly more so than acetaminophen—and it has a longer duration of action. Most ibuprofen preparations also taste better than those with acetaminophen. But ibuprofen has more potential for toxicity, especially for the kidneys.

Here's what we need to remember about acetaminophen: It's not recommended for infants younger than three months of age unless directed by a doctor, mainly because it might mask the presence of a potentially life-threatening infection. We have to be careful with the dosing of this medicine because too much can cause life-threatening liver problems. Follow the directions on the bottle or box, and you should be fine. If you've heard that a "loading dose" might be helpful (twice the regular dose), don't do it. It causes confusion and increases the risk of an overdose. Expect acetaminophen to begin working in 30 to 60 minutes and reach its peak effect in 3 to 4 hours. Its duration of action is anywhere between 4 and 6 hours. More than 80 percent of children will have their temperatures reduced by as much as 3.6 degrees.

Now, about ibuprofen. It shouldn't be given to an infant younger than six months of age unless your physician directs otherwise. Pay attention to the dosing of this drug as well. It's spaced out a little more, with at least 6 hours between doses. It begins working in less than an hour and has a peak effect in 3 to 4 hours. It's a little quicker than acetaminophen. The duration of action is 6 to 8 hours, and it lowers an elevated temperature to the same degree (see what we did there?) as acetaminophen.

### ✦ What about combining or alternating these medicines? Is that safe?

It might be safe, but we don't recommend it. Once again, fever is not a disease, and we don't want anyone obsessing with getting their child's temperature back to normal. Obsessing with that can lead to fever phobia (which might actually *be* a disease? Hmm). Anyway, the American Academy of Pediatrics advises against this practice, mainly because it can increase the possibility of inaccurate dosing. Pick your medicine and stick with it. If you start with acetaminophen and don't get the desired response, that would be the appropriate time to switch to ibuprofen. But don't alternate the two medicines.

The desired response from your child is that she's made to feel more comfortable. We're not recommending that you chase a fever until it's back to normal, only that you see that the medicine is causing your child to feel better. That's the goal with these drugs. As a caution, if the fever persists for more than four or five days, it's time to have your child examined. And if new symptoms appear—such as confusion, a stiff neck, a widespread rash, or decreased fluid intake—that can be an emergency. Get help.

Regarding external cooling methods, we generally don't recommend them. Sponging with alcohol should never be done because of the risk of adverse effects. And sponging with tepid water may help a little, but the effect is short-lived and your child won't like it.

So this is what you need to know: what causes a fever, when fever should be treated, and how to treat a fever. Fever phobia? Forget it.

And about putting your child in an ice bath...This would be a timely application of Luke 6:31: "Do to others as you would have them do to you."

> *"When dealing with a fever,*
> *treat the child and not the number."*
>
> A Professor of Pediatrics

# Febrile Seizures

✚ *Our one-year-old had what the ER doctor called*
*a "febrile seizure" last night. It scared us to death,*
*and we want to know how to keep this from*
*ever happening again. Can you help?*

We understand why you were scared. It's terrifying to watch your child having a seizure and feel powerless to stop it. And yes, we can help by explaining what we know about febrile seizures and by providing you with both some guidance and reassurance.

A febrile seizure refers to an episode that occurs in infancy or childhood, usually between the ages of six months and five years. It's associated with a fever but without evidence of anything serious going on in the brain. And it's *not* a form of epilepsy. For a seizure to be considered a febrile seizure, a few elements need to be present:

- an elevated temperature greater than 100.4
- the child older than six months and younger than five years
- no evidence of any brain infection or inflammation
- no evidence or history of any medical problems that might precipitate seizure activity (kidney disease, diabetes)
- no history of any seizure activity *without* a fever (epilepsy)

Essentially, this an episode of seizure activity in a child who has previously enjoyed good health.

Febrile seizures are divided into two categories: *simple* and *complex*.

This is important to know, because the type of seizure tells us a lot about what to expect in the future.

A *simple* febrile seizure is the more common of the two, and it's described as *generalized*. This means a child's body is jerking all over: arms, legs, and torso. It should last less than 15 minutes and should not happen again within a 24-hour period. Most of these seizures don't last more than 5 minutes, and some experts now use 10 minutes as the cut off. If it's your child, 5 minutes will seem like an eternity, but should this happen, keep an eye on the clock if you're calm enough to do so and note the duration. This will be important information for your physician.

A *complex* febrile seizure is defined as having a *focal* onset, which means the initial shaking starts in one arm, one leg, or one side of the body. It lasts longer than 15 minutes or occurs more than once in a 24-hour period. This type of febrile seizure is associated with a higher rate of recurrence and a slightly increased rate of epilepsy. We'll consider that in more detail a little later.

### ✚ I had never heard of a febrile seizure until our boy had one. How common is it?

This is the most common neurologic problem of infants and children, and it occurs in somewhere between 2 and 4 percent of children younger than five. That's about 4 in every 100 children. As a comparison, appendicitis occurs in 2 of every 10,000 children under age four. So this is common, and it affects boys slightly more than it does girls.

The risk factors include:

- *A young age.* This is an age-dependent problem because an infant's or toddler's brain is still developing and her seizure threshold (the point at which a fever occurs) is lower due to this immaturity. Most of these seizures will occur between 6 and 18 months of age.

- *A high fever.* We mentioned that the elevated temperature needs to be above 100.4 for a seizure to be febrile, but the usual temperatures we see are higher—somewhere around

103 or a little more. We were taught (as are most new physicians) that it's not the *height* of the temperature that's important but the *rate of rise* of the temperature. It turns out there's no evidence to support that view. The height of the fever is apparently the culprit. That will be important to keep in mind when we talk about how to prevent these seizures.

- *The presence of infection.* Most commonly, the infection causing this seizure will be a virus. (If it's caused by bacteria, we need to be more concerned about involvement of the brain or its lining.) But although several types of viruses cause most of these seizures, the type of virus isn't important. We're not going to have this information when your child comes into the ER or the doctor's office anyway.

- *Recent immunizations.* The risk for febrile seizure increases with certain vaccinations, including the ones for diphtheria, tetanus, and pertussis, as well as the MMR. This risk is minimal, though, and if a child has a febrile seizure following an immunization, most experts still recommend repeat vaccinations in the future because their benefits will still outweigh the risks.

- *Genetic predisposition.* We're not sure why, but there is a clear genetic predisposition for febrile seizures. That 4 percent incidence we noted earlier can be as high as 20 percent if a child's parents had febrile seizures. That same 20 percent is true for the sibling of a child who experiences one.

- *Prenatal exposure to nicotine and alcohol.* Smoking or vaping causes a slight increase in risk, but there's no apparent link to alcohol.

- *Allergic problems, such as eczema, allergic rhinitis, and even asthma.* This is an interesting association, but the increased risk is only minimal.

So what does this condition look like? Again, we know the age range, and it seems that the greatest risk is between the ages of 12 and 18 months. The majority of these seizures occur on the first day of illness, and sometimes they will be the first sign that a child is sick. And again, with a simple febrile seizure, we'll see a generalized shaking, with facial and respiratory muscles commonly involved. This can last up to 15 minutes, but, fortunately, the usual duration is only 3 to 4 minutes. Your child will quickly return to the normal baseline, though some confusion, agitation, or drowsiness might persist for a short time—up to 30 minutes or so. Longer than that and we will be concerned that something else is going on. When a seizure is over, the shaking stops and your child's eyes are closed, with his breathing slow and deep. If a child's eyes remain open and he's looking off to one side, the seizure probably hasn't stopped.

Complex seizures frequently occur in younger infants, and more so in those with developmental abnormalities or delays. Again, we'll see shaking in one arm or leg, and it will last more than 15 minutes. (This is another important reason to note the time of onset and duration of the seizure.)

### ✚ How will I know it's a seizure and not something else?

It will be hard to misidentify this problem. However, parents (and even physicians) can misinterpret the involuntary movements of shaking chills for a febrile seizure. The tip-off is that shaking chills are much more common and usually involve milder, more rhythmic movements around a joint (shoulders, elbows, wrists). We're not going to see facial involvement with a shaking chill, nor that of the respiratory muscles. Both sides of the body are usually involved at the same time, but there will not be a loss of consciousness. Another clue is that you should be able to stop the shaking of a chill by placing your hands on the involved joints/extremities of your child. You won't be able to do this with a febrile seizure.

### ✚ The ER doctor ordered a bunch of lab work and talked about doing a lumbar puncture. He was about to send

*our son to radiology to get a CT scan of his head,
but by then Jeffy was wide awake and running around
the room. We said no to that other stuff and took
him home. Did we do the right thing?*

It sounds like it. Remember the points that define this condition: age range, no evidence of any serious infection, some degree of fever, previous good health. If all those are present, coupled with a normal exam and quick return to the child's previous condition, we probably have the diagnosis. A lumbar puncture isn't needed in most well-appearing children. This procedure is indicated only with evidence or significant suspicion of meningitis, and a CT scan or MRI isn't required for children who quickly return to a normal baseline.

If you find yourself in the ER, the challenge might be engaging the doctor in a discussion about his desire to order invasive tests or substantial radiation exposure. A significant part of an ER doctor's motivation to order these can be based on a perceived medico-legal risk, which is unfortunate but true. This is just one more reason for you to know as much about this condition as possible.

Most of the time, a febrile seizure has ended on its own by the time the child gets to the doctor's office or ER and he's quickly returned to his normal baseline. If you called 9-1-1 and your boy was taken to the ER by ambulance, in some areas of the country, the paramedics might have given him antiseizure medication as a shot or through an IV line. That's okay, but the drowsiness caused by the medication will make evaluation a little more difficult and longer to achieve. But most of the time, a child stops seizing before EMS gets to the house, so the medication isn't needed. The good news is that with a simple febrile seizure and a normal exam, most children don't require hospitalization and can safely be sent home.

### ✛ But what if the seizure happens again?

Children with a febrile seizure do have an increased chance of having another one—maybe more than one. Here's what one large study found:

- The overall rate of recurrence is about 35 percent.

- The risk varies with age, from 50 to 65 percent in children younger than one year to as low as 20 percent in those older.

- Recurrences of 50 to 75 percent happen within one year of the initial seizure.

- Almost all recurrences occur within two years.

So recurrence is common—in about 1 in 3 children who have experienced them. Some factors, when present, can help us identify the child most at risk of recurrence:

- a young age at onset, closer to that six-month cutoff

- a history of febrile seizures in a parent or sibling

- a low degree of fever while in the doctor's office or ER

- a short duration of time between the onset of fever and the initial seizure[1]

If all four of these factors are present, the risk of the child having a recurrence is high, upwards of 70 percent. This compares with a risk of only 20 percent in the child who has none of the factors.

For children who have had one or more febrile seizures, the use of fever medication early on in a febrile illness may make the child feel better—even lower their temperature—but it doesn't appear to lower the incidence of another seizure. That's troubling and frustrating. As parents, we want to do something. We want to prevent another of those alarming and distressing events. It's still reasonable to give your child acetaminophen or ibuprofen if they're running a fever and are uncomfortable, but it's not going to stave off another seizure.

The good news is that most of the time (at least 66 percent), your child won't have a recurrence. The odds are even better if none of those risk factors noted above are present.

✚ *I read somewhere that a child who has a febrile seizure is more likely to develop epilepsy later on. Is that true?*

Probably. But the risk is only slightly more than those who never have a febrile seizure. The risk is greatest in those children who have complex febrile seizures (focal and prolonged) and those who have repeated seizures during the first 24 hours of the same illness. But again, the overall risk is small.

The bottom line is that febrile seizures are terrifying. We know that. And if your child has ever had one, you know that too. But be reassured: In its most common and simple form, this is frequently a one-and-done kind of problem. And if there's a recurrence, it can be managed. It doesn't mean your child is destined to have a lifelong seizure disorder.

Knowledge—it really helps with this one. It's reassuring.

*"It is the absence of facts that frightens people."*

Hilary Mantel

# 8

# Gastroenteritis and Dehydration

### ✛ How can I know if our child is dehydrated? And what can we do about it?

Dehydration is a common and serious problem for infants and young children. Fortunately, its onset is usually not subtle. It's marked by vomiting and diarrhea. The common denominator here is "volume depletion," which occurs when fluid is lost faster than it's taken in. The most common sites include the gastrointestinal tract (vomiting and diarrhea), the skin (burns and fever), and through the kidneys (diabetes and medications). "Insensible water losses," those that aren't readily apparent, occur through the skin when a child has a fever or increased sweating and through the process of breathing. Exhaled air contains water, and the faster a child breathes, the more water is lost.

> "Having children is like living in a frat house—nobody sleeps, everything's broken, and there's a lot of throwing up."
>
> **RAY ROMANO**

Young children are at an increased risk for a couple of reasons. They tend to have more episodes of gastroenteritis than do older children and adults, and because of their size, they're more vulnerable to those insensible losses. Importantly, infants and many toddlers aren't able to voice their sense of thirst and need for fluids.

Just because a child has vomited a couple of times doesn't necessarily mean she's dehydrated or headed that way. It's possible, though, and we need to assess the presence and degree of any dehydration. The best way to do this is to measure a change in weight from the normal baseline. That information isn't always going to be available. More often than not, when we ask parents what their child weighs, they look at each other with raised eyebrows. That's okay. Some of us can't remember our kids' middle names. If we do have an accurate baseline weight—measured in the past week or two—we can estimate a child's fluid deficit by using a simple formula: a loss of one pound represents a deficit of around 16 ounces.

For example, if your boy weighed 20 pounds and after two days of vomiting weighs 19 pounds (on the same scales and with the same clothing—or lack thereof), we can estimate that his one pound of weight loss represents a fluid deficit of around 16 ounces. That's important to know as we try to determine the presence and degree of dehydration and how we need to approach it.

Having a baseline weight doesn't happen very often. Kids grow, and their weight changes. It's hard to remember what they weigh one month to the next. One helpful strategy is to weigh your child at the onset of an episode of vomiting and diarrhea. Note it somewhere, and if the vomiting continues, we'll have a point of reference.

When a baseline weight isn't available, we can look for some other things to help determine the severity of dehydration:

- how long this has been going (the younger and smaller the child, the less tolerance for any significant fluid loss)

- a decrease in urine output (dry diapers for most of the day?)

- irritability or lethargy

- the child's heart rate  (the heart rate increases with dehydration)

- How fast and deep the child is breathing (remember those insensible water losses).

- The child's blood pressure reading (this helps us assess the overall fluid status because a low blood pressure is a red flag).

- "Skin turgor" (this has to do with the amount of fluid in the soft tissues). Normally, if you gently pinch the skin of the forearm, calf, or thigh, it will immediately return to a flat condition when the pinch is released. If there is significant dehydration and less fluid in the soft tissues, the skin flattens more slowly after that release. We call this "tenting," and it's cause for concern.

- How much blood is getting to the periphery—the child's fingers and toes. We can assess this by applying gentle pressure over a child's finger for five seconds. When released, the color should return to that finger in less than three seconds. More than that is abnormal and indicates an underlying process (such as dehydration) that is shunting blood away from less critical parts of the body, such as hands and feet. This is called the "capillary refill test." Try it when your child is healthy, and you'll see how it works.

As physicians, we try to determine the *degree* of dehydration by dividing it into three categories:

1. *Mild dehydration.* When we call dehydration mild, we're estimating a fluid loss of 3 to 5 percent of your child's total fluid volume. Frequently, this is based on the history you give us, because many of the signs noted above won't be present. There might be a reduced urine output, but that's not always easy to assess.

2. *Moderate dehydration.* For a moderate dehydration diagnosis, we're looking at a fluid loss of 6 to 9 percent. When this happens, those signs and symptoms we discussed will be apparent: low blood pressure, a rapid heart rate, dry mucous membranes (mouth and tongue), decreased skin turgor, irritability, and an increased capillary refill test—closer to three seconds or a little more.

3. *Severe dehydration.* A child with fluid losses of greater than

10 percent is a sick child. We'll see mottled extremities, lethargy, a markedly prolonged capillary refill test, low blood pressure, and a near shock-like appearance. This child needs to be in the hospital ASAP!

What you need to do is try to determine if a child with vomiting, diarrhea, and dehydration can be safely managed at home—in other words, the child has only mild (or maybe moderate) dehydration. (A severely dehydrated child should already be on the way to the ER.) These reliable indicators can help you assess a child with a 5 percent loss of fluid—the most commonly encountered state of dehydration and one that doesn't require hospitalization. The signs most frequently found with a 5 percent loss are a delayed capillary refill time (you know how to do that now), reduced skin turgor/tenting (you can do that too), and deeper than normal respirations (whether with an increased rate or not).

**✚ Okay, so now I know how to tell if my child is dehydrated, and our pediatrician has checked him out and agrees he's dehydrated, at least mildly. Now what? How can we safely manage him at home? We don't want to go to the ER unless it's absolutely necessary.**

You're right about the ER, so let's talk about how to handle this dehydration at home. It is difficult for even the most experienced physician to accurately differentiate between a child with mild dehydration and one with moderate dehydration. Thus, most experts will group these two into one treatment group, and that's what we're going to do.

The mainstay of treatment is "oral rehydration therapy" (ORT), using an "oral rehydration solution" (ORS). This is nothing new. It's been used in the developing world for decades and has saved the lives of countless children with life-threatening diarrheal disease.

Let's start with the ORS. Most of us are familiar with Pedialyte—a rehydrating solution readily available in stores. Others are out there, but Pedialyte has a long track record of success and ease of use. The composition of any ORS is important, and a couple of key points are crucial. The concentrations of glucose and sodium need to be comparable. Too much glucose will cause a problem, and too little sodium will do the same. Pedialyte is a balanced solution and gives a child what she needs.

Parents have tried a lot of different fluids for their dehydrated child, including soda, sports drinks, and fruit juices. But these have too much sugar and will increase diarrhea and dehydration. Then there's chicken soup and chicken broth, but they have way too much sodium, which will also cause an increase in diarrhea and create electrolyte problems. It's not uncommon for parents to find a recipe for an ORS on the internet and try to mix up a batch at home. That's fraught with a lot of potential problems and errors in mixing. There's too much at stake to take this kind of chance.

### ✚ Wait a minute.
### You're telling me Pedialyte is as good as an IV?

That's what we're saying, and that's what the evidence shows, for any balanced ORS. Remember, we're not dealing with severe dehydration, which should not be treated at home.

Once we decide on an ORS, treatment begins in two phases:

1. *The "rehydration phase."* After estimating the child's fluid deficit—as an example, that 5 percent loss we talked about earlier—the key is to offer him small amounts of the ORS every one or two minutes by spoon or syringe, usually 5 ml (one teaspoon). At this rate, you can give a child 150 to 300 ml in an hour (300 ml would be about 10 ounces). The goal is to replace the deficit as quickly as possible, preferably over three to four hours, without overloading a child's stomach. A reasonable target is to give the child with mild/moderate dehydration about an ounce per pound of body weight over that time frame. We sometimes get questions about breastfeeding and whether it should be stopped during this part of the process. The

answer is no, both during this phase of treatment and through the next.

2. *The "maintenance phase."* Now that we've corrected our deficit, we want to maintain our fluid status. We can cut back a little on the amount of ORS, depending on the frequency of any ongoing diarrhea. The important thing is to begin feeding the child with an age-appropriate and unrestricted diet. Basically, she can eat what she normally eats. Some doctors do recommend limiting the fat content of meals and snacks, as do we, especially if the diarrhea continues. At this point, and with mild gastroenteritis, you can try diluted apple juice (half strength) as a maintenance fluid if your child likes that better than the Pedialyte or another ORS.

This might sound too complicated, but it's not. And it works. You'll know you're making progress when your child's activity level improves, she starts wetting her diapers, and her respirations and heart rate slow down. Stay in close contact with your pediatrician's office and let them know about any concerns you have or if your child isn't progressing as you would expect.

### ✚ We're going to follow your advice, but what can we give our child for the vomiting and diarrhea?

Let's talk for a moment about gastroenteritis and what we can expect. Gastroenteritis is defined by an increased stool frequency—three or more loose or watery stools in 24 hours or a number of such stools that exceeds your child's usual number of daily bowel movements by two or more. This might last as long as a week, but no longer than two weeks, and it might or might not be accompanied by vomiting or fever. This isn't going to stop overnight, so be patient.

As we previously noted, diet is important, with the resumption of what your child normally eats as quickly as possible. Again, we recommend limiting fatty foods and also those with high levels of simple sugars. Yogurt, fruits, vegetables, complex carbohydrates, and lean meats are fine. It seems that the oft-recommended "BRAT" diet (bananas, rice, applesauce, and toast) is too restrictive, not nutritionally optimal, and unneeded. Regarding reducing lactose-containing foods (milk and milk products), it appears that doing so might have some benefit—possibly reducing the duration of diarrhea by almost a day. The evidence is not overwhelming, but the reduction is worth a try.

> "Laughter is always the best medicine...unless you have diarrhea."
>
> **AUTHOR UNKNOWN**

When we or our children are sick, we want to reach for *something*—some familiar medication or remedy, maybe a prescription medicine in our cabinet. When the problem is vomiting or diarrhea, we do the same thing, probably quicker. But what works and what's safe?

First, we need to keep in mind that viral gastroenteritis (the most common cause of this problem) is self-limited. It's going to go away on its own. Frequently used antidiarrheal agents should *not* be routinely used with our children. There is no evidence that they work, and they might have significant side effects. These agents include the antimotility drugs, such as Lomotil and Imodium. The thought here is that by slowing down intestinal motility, we're allowing the infectious bugs to remain in the GI tract for a longer period of time. We know this is true for bacterial infections, and it might also be true for viruses.

Medications that reduce the movement of fluid into the intestines have been used for decades. Pepto-Bismol and Kaopectate are a couple of these medications, but they're not recommended for children. The bismuth contained in them causes the stool to turn black—a frequent precipitant of a 3:00 a.m. phone call to your doctor. Kaopectate is another remedy that's been around for a long time. It's basically clay, and it's supposed to bind stuff in your child's gut. Once again, there's no valid evidence that it works.

When it comes to vomiting, we're *really* motivated to do something for our children. It's frightening for them and alarming for us. We have a safe and effective medicine for this—ondansetron (Zofran)—and it can be used in children older than six months if there's evidence of dehydration or if the vomiting is interfering with oral rehydration therapy. This is a prescription medication, and it comes in a handy orally dissolving wafer. It has few side effects (but an increased risk of diarrhea with multiple doses), and it's been proven to reduce the need for IV therapy. A few medications should *not* be used for vomiting. They include Phenergan, Compazine, Benadryl, and Domperidone. The potential side effects and risks far outweigh any possible benefit to your child.

> "Most of the common infections— colds, flu, diarrhea— you get environmentally transmitted either in the air or on surfaces you touch. I think people underrate surfaces."
>
> **CHARLES P. GERBA**

We've been hearing a lot about probiotics and prebiotics and how they're good for just about everything. When it comes to the treatment of diarrhea, the jury is still out. They may be beneficial, and they shouldn't cause any harm, but if you decide to use one, it should probably be a combination product (lactobacillus, inulin, and others) and started early in the course of the gastroenteritis.

### ✚ How can we keep gastroenteritis from spreading in our home, and when can our children go back to day care or school?

Good luck with keeping gastroenteritis contained. Viral gastroenteritis is highly contagious, and you have to be vigilant. Frequent handwashing with soap and water is effective, but be aware that alcohol-based hand sanitizers don't work very well for the *norovirus*—the most commonly found virus in children who have to be admitted to the hospital for dehydration. The *rotavirus* is another common cause, but our children should be vaccinated against it. That immunization is important, because this virus is the leading cause of death worldwide in children with infectious gastroenteritis.

Wherever you change your child's diapers should be far away from where any food is prepared or consumed, and the diapers need to be disposed of immediately in some kind of bag and moved outside the house. Sounds obvious, but it doesn't always happen. The changing area should be wiped down, but, remember, alcohol won't always be effective. A diluted bleach solution works best.

The question of when a child can return to school or day care is a good one. Obviously, the diarrhea and vomiting needs to have stopped, but for how long?

The American Academy of Pediatrics gives us the following advice:

> Children with diarrhea may return to childcare or school provided that
>
> - stools are contained in the diaper (for infants),
> - the child has no accidents (older children), and
> - stool frequency is less than two stools greater than the child's normal stool frequency.[1]

Regarding vomiting, if your child has endured two or more episodes in the previous 24 hours, he shouldn't return to school. You'll need to wait until this has resolved.

The National Institute for Health and Care Excellence (NICE) has more restrictive recommendations. They advise that children be excluded from childcare or school for at least 48 hours after the last episode of vomiting or diarrhea. These more restrictive recommendations are more protective and pose less risk to other children. Your day care or school might have their own guidelines, but these are reasonable strategies.

Whew! That's a lot of information, but this is a common problem and something we're all going to face as parents. We have effective ways to deal with gastroenteritis and dehydration, and we need to be prepared.

*"Prepare and prevent,*
*don't repair and repent."*

Author Unknown

# 9

# Sleep

### ✚ How much sleep does my child need?

That's a great question, and even though you didn't mention how old your child is, every parent needs to have a good understanding about how much sleep children need at any age. Children of different ages need different amounts of sleep.

Here are the recommendations from the American Academy of Sleep Medicine (AASM) and endorsed by the American Academy of Pediatrics (AAP):

| Age Group | Recommended Sleep Time |
| --- | --- |
| Infants up to 4 months | 18 or more hours |
| Infants 4 to 12 months | 12 to 16 hours (including naps) |
| Infants 1 to 2 years | 11 to 14 hours (including naps) |
| Children 3 to 5 years | 10 to 13 hours (including naps) |
| Children 6 to 12 years | 9 to 12 hours |
| Teens 13 to 18 years | 8 to 10 hours[1] |

Interesting stuff. If you have a teenager, do you think they're getting eight hours of sleep each night? Probably not, and for a couple of reasons. First, sleep patterns and average lengths of sleep have progressively declined over the past few decades, probably reflecting how our children entertain themselves with the use of electronic gadgets and games. Second, sleep times for children in the United States tend to be shorter than those in Australian and European children.[2] This is especially true on weekdays. It is estimated that more than 60 percent of US adolescents get less than seven hours of sleep on weekday nights.[3] This is a lot less than the recommended eight to ten hours for this age group. Not sure how much sleep your nine-year-old is getting? Or your fourteen-year-old? You're not alone. Tweens and teens want their privacy. But this is important, and we need to pay attention. If you don't know where your child fits on that table, you need to figure it out.

### ✚ How can I tell if my child isn't getting enough sleep? Is it a big deal if she isn't?

It is a big deal, and here's why: Sleep deficiency, whatever the cause, results in reduced alertness, impaired performance, and negative consequences for health. These problems are largely behavioral, performance in nature, and more readily apparent in children than in adults. This is true for all of us, but we're going to consider how it affects our children.

An expected first sign of sleep deficiency is a decrease in attention and reaction time. For school-aged children, this can be manifested by their inability to respond quickly and accurately to a host of things. At school, this can include the inability to perform well on computerized testing. They may be able to arrive at a correct answer, but it takes them longer. Other concerns are an impairment in activities that require speed and accuracy, such as driving a car, taking a standardized test, or even crossing a busy highway. That should scare us.

Lack of sleep also results in an impairment of complex cognitive functions. These functions can include decision making, selective attention, judgment, problem solving, multitasking, and time management. The list goes on, and these are obviously important for a child's well-being and successful development on many levels.

Academic performance is affected by sleep deprivation, and not in a good way. With greater lack of sleep, we see worsening academic success and school performance. This is obviously reflected in poor grades but also with a loss of motivation to succeed, a poor self-image, and tension between student and teacher.

Sleep is known to be a crucial and active part of the process of organizing our memory. Putting a book under our pillow is not going to help us learn something, but adequate sleep will help us organize and retain memories of what we've *just* learned. This is true for learning about specific facts but also for motor skills and emotional processing. If you have a toddler, what is the importance of her afternoon nap? It seems that a daytime nap will help her consolidate learning memories and motor skill learning. Don't rush to eliminate this part of her day.

> "People who say they sleep like a baby usually don't have one."
>
> **LEO J. BURKE**

Sleep deprivation has a significant and consistent impact on emotional and behavioral reactions. We see increased irritability, moodiness, depression, and anger. (Sounds like a typical teenager, doesn't it? But this is worse.) Of significant concern is an increase in suicidal thoughts among children with inadequate or disrupted sleep.

So we can be aware of, look for, and then try to improve a lot of things. The first step is to get a handle on the amount of sleep your child is getting, especially your teenager. If it doesn't match the recommendations, make some changes. Lights out at a specific time is a good place to start—and that means all electronic devices off too. Only a little more sleep can make a big difference. In fact, as little as 30 minutes of additional sleep can provide measurable increases in school performance and behavior. Thirty minutes. That's not much, but it will take a consistent effort to get there.

### ✚ My 14-year-old likes to catch up on his sleep on the weekend. Isn't that okay?

Nope. It might be hurting rather than helping. Sleep patterns should be consistent, regardless of the day of the week. You might have heard of circadian rhythms. This is an internal 24-hour clock that tells us when to sleep, when to wake up, and even when to eat. There's some variation among individuals, but this is usually associated with light and dark, daytime and nighttime. It can change some as we age, but it's largely consistent.

When we disrupt this cycle, bad things happen. Jet lag is a prime example. Your teenager's oversleeping on the weekend (sometimes referred to as "weekend oversleep"—imagine that) can disrupt their circadian rhythm, compounding an already significant problem. The answer is to encourage a consistent and adequate sleep pattern, and it should start when your child is an infant. If that time has passed, make the right changes now. Tonight.

*"The only thing worth stealing is a kiss from a sleeping child."*

J.H. Oldham

## 10

# Behavioral Insomnia

✚ *Bedtime with our four-year-old has become Armageddon.*
*How can we get her to go to bed without*
*wearing all of us out?*

Bedtime battles. You're not alone. Somewhere between 20 and 30 percent of all children have some form of childhood insomnia. This can be the result of a medical issue, such as obstructive sleep apnea (yes, young children can develop this as well as adults), medications, pain, and anxiety, as well as developmental issues. But far and away, the most common cause of sleep disturbances in children is a "behavioral sleep problem." This can come in various forms, but the most common are bedtime resistance/refusal, delayed sleep onset, and nighttime awakenings. What can make these challenging—as if they weren't already challenging enough—is that some of these causes can coexist.

A behavioral sleep problem is most common in young children from birth to five years of age, but it can persist into middle childhood and adolescence. By definition, for your child to have a "sleep disorder," the symptoms need to occur at least three times a week and persist for at least three months. In addition, there has to be some degree of dysfunction in the child, parents, and/or family.

Bedtime resistance sounds straightforward. Every parent has experienced the child who refuses to go to bed, and we've heard a lot of different and imaginative excuses from that child. Some degree of this is common, probably normal, but it should be a passing problem. When it persists, difficulties arise.

Delayed sleep onset is just what it says—a prolonged amount of time before your child falls asleep. There is no specific time frame here, but 15 to 30 minutes is a reasonable expectation.

Prolonged nighttime awakening is frequently the first problem we encounter, and it can easily result in insufficient sleep. Children experience a normal 60- to 90-minute cycling of specific types of sleep (REM as an example), and a certain amount of arousal occurs at the end of each cycle. If a child wakes up, he or she might not be able to go back to sleep. This is the 3:00 a.m. crying that rouses the entire house or the toddler who climbs out of her bed and into yours.

These behavioral problems are generally caused by one of two things. The first is "sleep-onset associations." The infant or child has learned to fall asleep only when a specific routine takes place, like rocking until he's asleep or being fed right before sleep. He briefly wakes during the night, which is normal, but without anyone to rock or feed him. He's unable to self-soothe and wants his usual routine—loudly announced by his crying or getting out of bed. We'll look at effective ways to deal with this behavior a little later.

The other factor that causes these behavioral problems is—you guessed it—inadequate or ineffective parenting. Here we see most of the verbal protests, active resistance, or repeated demands for stories or for the parent's presence. The disorder usually develops from our unwillingness or inability to set and keep bedtime rules. First-time parents are especially at risk, but so are those of us with much more experience and who should know better. It's easy to fall into a routine that is harmful to your child, to you, and to the rest of the family.

### ✚ But all of my four children have experienced problems with their sleeping. It must be genetic.

Hmm. All of your children? The problem might not be in their genes. We know that only about 25 percent of childhood sleep disorders are "intrinsic"—genetically influenced. The remainder and vast majority are because of "extrinsic" factors, such as parenting techniques, home environment (sharing of bedrooms, a bedroom's temperature), and emotional stress in the home.

So given that the majority of children's sleep disorders are behavioral and that the majority of those exist because of extrinsic factors, let's look at some proven ways to resolve these problems. And they *can* be resolved.

Parents will see significant improvement in more than 80 percent of children with the use of these simple techniques, and no study shows any detrimental effects. Once we've addressed and improved the sleep disorder, other positive things start to happen as well, such as better daytime behavior, less crying and irritability, and enhanced overall emotional well-being. That's true for our children, and it's true for everyone in the house.

Now for those simple techniques, divided into several types of intervention.

## Bedtime Routines

A bedtime routine needs to be consistent and should take 20 to 40 minutes. It's okay to include several activities during this time, such as taking a bath, dressing in pajamas, and reading a story or two. The key is for any bedtime activity to be soothing and with no television or electronic devices. It's also okay to provide a comforting object, such as a blanket or toy. This can help your child fall asleep. It can also provide a source of comfort or self-soothing should she wake up during the night. And here's an important point: Your children should be put to bed when they're still awake but drowsy. This will help reduce the need/demand for your presence as they fall asleep.

## Systematic Ignoring

Systematic ignoring addresses the problem of your child's demanding that you stay in the room until they fall asleep. They also do this when they wake up in the middle of the night, and there are two ways to deal with it. The first is to let them cry it out. This works and does no harm. But some parents, especially those with a first child, aren't able to do this. That's all right. We can accomplish the same goal by gradually weaning children of a parent's presence in their bedroom.

Again, it starts with putting your child to bed when drowsy but awake and waiting for progressively longer periods of time to check on him or her. When checking, the time spent needs to be brief—only a minute or two—and with minimal contact. A pat on the shoulder is fine, but avoid picking them up and cuddling them. That only reinforces the behavior you're trying to alter. It's a step backward.

## Strategic Napping

This is where you need to know the recommended sleep requirements for your infant or older child. We looked at that in a previous chapter, and the requirements include both nighttime sleep and napping. As a general rule, though, children need at least four hours between sleep periods to be able to fall asleep again. A late afternoon nap, extending into the early evening, can disrupt their normal routine.

This is a good time to consider your child's sleep window. Again, you need to know the amount of recommended sleep based on age. For example, a four-year-old needs ten to thirteen hours of sleep each day, including naps. If your daughter routinely takes a two- or three-hour nap in the afternoon, you'll need to match her in-bed time at night to her remaining sleep requirement. That should be somewhere between nine and ten hours. If we put children in bed and expect them to stay there for twelve hours, we've created a mismatch. They will either take longer going to sleep or wake up earlier, both of which can be problematic. It's not rocket science, but it's important. Know your child's sleep requirement.

## Positive Reinforcement

It's true that you can catch more flies with honey than with vinegar, but who wants to catch flies? We want our children to go to bed peacefully, get a good night's sleep, and wake up alert and in a good mood. Positive reinforcement in the form of a reward is effective and acceptable. We need to keep in mind that any such reward needs to be immediate (the next morning), something obtainable (matching the desired behavior to something your child can do), and something that interests and motivates him. Multiple small rewards seem to be more effective than a few larger ones.

With all that in mind, here are our pointers for your child's healthy sleep:

- Have a set bedtime and routine and be consistent.

- Make both weekday and weekend bedtimes consistent, with no more than one hour of variance.

- Don't send your child to bed hungry. A big meal just before sleep can be a problem, but a protein-rich snack will help.

- Make the hour before bed a shared and meaningful "quiet time." (Besides, these years and opportunities will pass all too quickly.)

- Eliminate television, computer games, smartphones, or high-energy activities for at least an hour before bed—preferably more. (Your child's bedroom shouldn't have a TV in it!)

- As your child grows older—and the same applies for you—avoid caffeine in any form for several hours before bedtime. The experts tell us six hours to be safe.

- Make sure your child is getting plenty of exercise, preferably outdoors, weather permitting.

- Make sure your child's bedroom is cool enough. It appears that 70 degrees or less provides the best temperature environment.

- Make sure the room is quiet and dark. A fan or sound machine can provide soothing, ambient background noise. If a night-light is needed, make sure it's not too bright.

- Don't use your child's bedroom for any form of punishment or time-out.

Keep these pointers in mind, map out an appropriate strategy, and stick with it. It won't happen overnight, but your child's quality of sleep will improve, and everyone will rest a little easier.

And about Armageddon…Remember who wins.

> *"There are two philosophies when it comes*
> *to getting young children to sleep.*
> *There is 'sleep training,' which basically involves*
> *putting your kids to bed and listening to them scream all night;*
> *or there is 'attachment,'*
> *which essentially involves lying down with your kids,*
> *cuddling them, and then listening to them scream all night."*

Jim Gaffigan

# 11

# Night Terrors and Nightmares

✚ *Is there a difference between night terrors and nightmares?*
*And what can we do about them?*

It's midnight, and you and your husband are sound asleep when a bloodcurdling scream jars you awake. Then you hear the sound of footsteps pounding down the hallway toward your bedroom. Heart racing, your breath coming in gasps, you frantically reach for your bedside lamp and switch it on.

Your two older children run into the room and clamber onto your bed.

"Johnny's having another nightmare! Do something, Mama!"

If you're a parent, you've probably been here—startled from sleep, trying to get your bearings, wondering what to do.

Night terrors and nightmares are in the same family of "parasomnias"—disorders that intrude on normal sleep. But they manifest themselves in different ways and have different treatment techniques.

A night terror is an episode where a child wakes suddenly from sleep and acts very upset. She might be sweating, trembling, breathing fast, or experiencing a bounding heartbeat. The episode will usually last 10 to 20 minutes, and nothing you do will calm them down. A couple of precipitating factors can be having a fever and experiencing chronic sleep deficiency for a variety of reasons. A night terror usually occurs during the first few hours of sleep, in contrast to a nightmare, which happens during the second half of sleep. And the child will usually go back to sleep after night terrors and not remember anything of the event in the morning.

A nightmare is a scary, frightening, or upsetting dream that can wake your child from sleep just as it does for adults. We're not sure why we experience nightmares, but when your child is awakened from one, it's difficult for him to go back to sleep. And he probably will remember the dream in the morning.

Night terrors and nightmares can be a little difficult to tell apart. Remember that night terrors usually occur in the first part of the night and that your child, once the episode is over (don't try to wake them up!), can be consoled and will go back to sleep. After a nightmare, your child will have trouble going back to sleep. One thing that might help calm him and get him to doze off again is to gently reassure him that what he just experienced was only a dream and not real. Some experts suggest drawing a picture of the dream or writing about it. That takes a little time, but it should make the dream less scary, maybe even funny. You can also help your child come up with an alternative ending for the dream—something happy and magical.

Because night terrors usually occur during the first part of the night, you might be able to identify a pattern, a time when they're most common—say, 11:30 to midnight. If that's the case, you can try "scheduled awakening." Gently wake your child 15 to 20 minutes before the anticipated event, but then let them go back to sleep in only a few minutes and see if it works.

From a medical standpoint, we would worry about night terrors only if they become nightly occurrences, disrupting the entire household, or your child has experienced physical changes that might be significant. These would include bed-wetting (if they previously were dry at night), loud snoring or gasping during sleep (obstructive sleep apnea is possible, but unusual in children), and any seizure activity or anything that looks like it might be a seizure. Any of those symptoms would be emergent.

As we've noted before, sufficient and good-quality sleep is important for all of us, especially our children. Make sure you know the recommended amount of sleep for your child, set a bedtime and abide by it, and develop a calming and quiet routine before sleep. Doing all of these things might not eliminate night terrors and nightmares, but they will help.

> *"From ghoulies and ghosties and long leggedy beasties*
> *and things that go bump in the night,*
> *Good Lord, deliver us!"*
>
> Old Scottish Saying

## 12

# Bed-Wetting

✛ *Our six-year-old wets the bed just about every night.*
*We've tried everything, and nothing works. Help!*

I f it makes you feel any better, you're not alone. Just remember the number 15. At age six, 15 percent of children will still be wetting the bed. Every year after that, 15 percent of these children will stop wetting the bed, and by age 15, this problem will almost always have resolved. But none of us want to wait until our child is a teenager before we stop changing wet sheets in the middle of the night. We want to address this problem as soon as possible.

The good news is, yes, we can help. Let's start with defining this condition.

"Nocturnal enuresis" (NE) refers to discrete episodes of urinary incontinence during sleep in children more than five years of age. That age is important because children younger than five haven't sufficiently matured (brain and bladder) to consistently stay dry at night. If your child stopped wetting the bed at age three, give thanks. That would be the exception. If he's still wetting the bed at four, that would be the rule. We need to stress this point: Don't expect or demand too much from your child. Keep the age of five in mind.

> "Nature, time, and patience are three great physicians."
>
> **HENRY GEORGE BOHN**

Eighty percent of the time, we'll be dealing with a simple form of NE. There's a complex form as well, and we need to know a few things about that because some frequently underlying problems must be diagnosed and treated before the NE can be addressed. Your child's NE is *not* simple if the following symptoms are present:

- a daytime loss of urinary control
- An increased frequency of urination (eight or more times a day) or a decreased frequency (three times or fewer). The average child voids around five to six times a day.
- a weak urinary stream
- hesitancy
- a feeling of incomplete bladder emptying
- lower abdominal or genital pain
- post-voiding dribbling
- straining to urinate
- Weight loss and an increase in the frequency of urination (this might be the first manifestation of diabetes).

If these symptoms are present, it's a different ball game, and your physician will adjust the approach accordingly. Our focus here is on *simple* NE.

We'll start with what we know about normal bladder maturation. During the first three years of life, bladder capacity consistently increases, and the development of bladder control follows a predictable course. First, your child becomes aware of bladder filling, at least during the day. This begins to happen around age three and is usually well developed by age four. At the same time, kids are learning to control the muscles that close and open the bladder outlet. All of this should come together by the age of five or six, at which time this daytime awareness extends through the night. Girls seem to mature faster here, and that's probably why more males are affected with NE than females.

Things can go wrong with this maturational journey, causing delays and frustration. Some of these include sleep disturbances, the production of a large amount of urine during the night, genetics (more about that in a minute), and even constipation.

### ✚ What about a small bladder?
### My grandmother always said that was my problem.

Hmm. We need to talk about your grandmother. But first, let's consider this idea of a small bladder or small bladder capacity. At birth, the normal bladder volume is about 60 milliliters (2 ounces). With each passing year, this volume increases by about an ounce, so that at age five, your child's bladder capacity is around 6 or 7 ounces. This can be important because a smaller bladder can lead to more frequent voiding during the day and a decreased ability to hold urine during the night. A small bladder isn't a common problem, but it can be measured if we hit a roadblock with treatment.

Now back to your grandmother. If she was referring to *your* problem with bed-wetting, that's interesting. Genetics play an important role with NE, with a strong tendency of it developing in the children of parents who had the problem themselves. If one parent has a history of NE, then half of their children will have it. If both parents were affected, then up to 75 percent of their children will be affected. It's probably too late to put something like that in your prenuptial agreement, but it's certainly something to keep in mind as your family expands.

There's also the issue of a child being a heavy sleeper. It turns out this can be an important factor. Central to NE is the child's inability to awaken to the normal stimulation to void. Parents will report this as "Johnny sleeps like a log, and it's hard to wake him up." It's this difficulty with arousal from sleep that separates a child with NE from one who senses the need to void and gets up in the middle of the night.

Earlier, we mentioned that constipation can be a problem and delay the bladder maturation process. If constipation isn't recognized and treated, the chances of improving the NE fall to just about zero. On the other hand, if the constipation is corrected, sometimes the NE will go away on its own. You'll need to observe, ask questions, and keep this potential and common problem in mind.

If you take your child to a doctor about this problem, in addition to obtaining a thorough history and performing a physical exam, she'll consider all of these things before deciding on a treatment plan. There's one more final hurdle to cross, and that has to do with the child's interest in addressing this problem. Obviously, this is of concern to you, your spouse, and probably other family members. But is it of concern to your child? If he doesn't see bed-wetting as a problem or isn't interested in addressing it, the prudent decision is to wait to address it. This situation is not going to get better unless your child wants it to.

Give it six to eight more months, and then address it again. The NE might very well disappear during that time. If not, some degree of maturation will have taken place, and treatment will have a better chance of success. But only if the interest is there.

### ✚ It might not be a problem for my boy, but it's a problem for the rest of us. We need to do something.

You *are* doing something. You're talking about NE and learning about it. We understand your frustration, but as with most things pediatric, a large dose of patience is necessary. Frustration quickly leads to anger and then to poor decisions. This is not your child's fault, and punishment should *never* be a part of your response. No good will ever come of it, but it seems that as many as 1 in 3 parents punish their child for bed-wetting—sometimes with physical abuse. Don't allow yourself to be in that number.

As we establish our treatment plan, two important things need to happen. First, start an "elimination diary" for your child. How many times does she void each day? How many bowel movements does she have (with some description of size and consistency)? How much fluid does she consume, and with what types of drinks? Caffeine can be part of this problem and needs to be significantly reduced or eliminated. Having this information provides a benchmark, and at times it points to the cause of the problem (drinking too much liquid in the evening). As another general rule, two-thirds of your child's fluid intake should occur before the end of the school day, with only one-third consumed in the evening and none during the hour or so before bed.

The second thing is to decide on the goal(s) of treatment. What do you want to see happen? This is important and needs input from everyone in the family, including your child. Some goals might be to

- reduce the number of wet nights,
- gain the ability to stay dry on specific occasions (spending the night with a friend),
- reduce the impact of NE on the family, or
- eliminate NE altogether.

Whatever the goal, it will need to be clearly defined, uniformly agreed upon, and achievable.

Now we're ready to consider the management of NE and decide on what course of action is best for your child and your family. Every plan needs to include education about the nature of this problem, as well as reassuring everyone involved that the chance of success and resolution of NE is high. We need to be optimistic that this is going to get better because...well, it's going to get better. At the same time, we need to stress the importance of patience.

We like the idea of incorporating motivational therapy in any treatment plan we develop. Your child should be rewarded in some small but meaningful way when he has a dry night. Be consistent, don't overdo it, and don't withhold the reward because of some other, unrelated problem.

Both of these two first-line treatments for NE have a good track record for effectiveness and safety.

## An Enuresis Alarm

An enuresis alarm is the most effective long-term therapy for NE. It's composed of a sensor that's placed in your child's undergarments or on a bed pad and an alarm that is either audible or that vibrates. It goes off when your child—let's say a boy—wets the bed. We prefer the audible alarm because then *you* know when it goes off. Here's the process:

- Your child wets, the alarm goes off, and he turns off the alarm. (Only the child should turn off the alarm.)
- You go to his room and make sure he's fully awake.
- Your child finishes voiding in the toilet.

- He returns to the bedroom and changes the bedding and his underwear. It's important for him to change the bedding himself as well. (An extra set of bedding should be kept nearby, where it can be easily found at three o'clock in the morning.)
- Your child wipes down the sensor and replaces it.
- He resets the alarm and goes back to bed.

Use of the alarm will be successful in as many as two-thirds of children. Early signs of success/response will be smaller wet patches, your child waking each time to the alarm, fewer alarms per night, the alarm going off later in the night, and fewer wet nights. It's thought that the alarm works through a conditioning process. The child learns to awaken or inhibit bladder contraction as he responds to the feelings present before wetting. Whatever the reason, this works. We recommend its use for at least two to three months. If effective, it should be continued until at least 14 consecutive dry nights have been achieved. At that point, you can try stopping. If there's a relapse, start again. A significant number of children will experience success the *second* time around.

Take a look at these websites to get a better idea of what we're talking about:

- Nighthawk Bedwetting Alarm—www.nighthawkbedwetting.com
- NiteTrain'R Bedwetting Alarm and Pads—www.nitetrainr.com
- SleepDry Alarm—www.sleepdryalarm.com

## Desmopressin (DMP)

This drug works by reducing the amount of urine produced overnight, and it has a long record of successful use and safety. The success rate can be up to 40 percent, and while easier to use than the alarm, it can be expensive, and the relapse rate is a little higher. You'll see the same positive responses as with the alarm, only a little quicker. There's a spray available, but it's not recommended, so stick with the pill.

While safe to use nightly, many guidelines suggest stopping the medicine every three months to see if it's still needed and to allow your child some time off the medication. DMP works best when NE has started to decrease in frequency (not every night) and can be safely used until the bed-wetting has completely been controlled. This is one of those drugs that needs to be tapered to stop using it. Reduce the nightly dose in half for two weeks, then quit. An important benefit of this drug is that once its effectiveness has been established, it can be used periodically when your child is going to spend the night (or a couple of nights) somewhere other than home. He can simply take the medication on the nights away.

Other treatments are out there, including different medications and even acupuncture, but nothing works as well as the two options we've presented. And one of these should be the first you try. It will be a matter of personal preference for you, your family, and your child.

For more information, we recommend a couple of good sources:

- The American Academy of Pediatrics—AAP.org
- The International Children's Continence Society—i-c-c-s. org

There's help for NE, and it will get better. Just remember the rule of 15.

*"The two most powerful warriors*
*are patience and time."*

Leo Tolstoy

# 13

# Sticks and Stones...and Collarbones

*Our two-year-old nephew fell and broke his wrist. I told my sister to be thankful it wasn't fractured. I'm right, aren't I?*

"Mrs. Dagenhart, why don't you bring Noah over here and we'll take a look at his X-rays."

I flipped the switch of the view box, backlighting the films of the three-year-old's wrist. Mrs. Dagenhart walked up behind me, carrying her young son.

"I know most parents aren't used to looking at X-rays," I told her, pointing to a buckled area in one of the bones of his wrist, "but that's where he broke it."

She leaned closer, peering at the film. "Oh good, Dr. Lesslie. At least it's not fractured."

*Say what?* Broken, fractured, cracked...They're all the same thing, and they all have the same implications.

We encounter another common misconception on an almost daily basis.

"Andrew fell at the skating rink and hurt his arm. We wanted to get it X-rayed, but there's probably nothing wrong since he can move it."

Not so fast. Just because someone can move an injured finger, wrist, arm, or ankle doesn't mean it's not broken. Movement doesn't mean anything, though this medical wisdom is ingrained in many of us. Just like "starve a cold and feed a fever." Or is it "feed a cold and starve a fever"?

Pediatric bones and joints pose a unique set of problems and potential pitfalls. The good news is that most boney injuries in children do very well with the right attention and treatment. Kids heal quickly, and this includes their bones. As an example, a fractured wrist in a 40-year-old will take four to six weeks to resolve, assuming there is good alignment and immobilization. A four-year-old's wrist will heal in as little as three weeks, again with adequate immobilization. And the healing is more complete, with less chance of resultant arthritis or limitation of movement. For instance, if I saw that 40-year-old ten years from now with another hand or forearm injury, I would probably ask him, "When did you break your wrist?" His bone might have completely healed, but you would forever be able to tell where it was broken. Not so with the four-year-old. In as little as a year, you wouldn't be able to find the site, its remodeling having resolved any telltale sign.

This is interesting stuff, and important. Kids' fractures usually do well if they are properly diagnosed and treated.

Here's another significant orthopedic term for the parents of young children: a greenstick fracture. Maybe you've heard that or a buckle or torus fracture. This usually occurs in any of a child's long bones (forearm, humerus, lower leg), and conceptually it's more the stress/bending of a bone rather than a complete break. If you or I fell on ice and landed on our outstretched hand, we would probably snap one of the bones in our wrist—usually the radius. A child might also slip and fall, land on his wrist or hand, and that bone would be "broken" but not in two.

Think of holding a small limb from a dogwood tree and bending it. Rather than cracking apart like an old, dry stick would, it bends and frays but doesn't completely separate. One side usually remains intact. That's what frequently happens with a child's bone. It's the reason they heal so quickly. Again, it has to be diagnosed and treated appropriately, and sometimes the bone must be manipulated a little to make sure the alignment is corrected, but usually the key for most of these injuries is immobilization and a little time.

We'll consider several important pediatric orthopedic issues, but right now let's take a look at one of the most common boney problems we encounter and what you need to know about it.

An anxious mother told me, "Ricky and his brother were on their trampoline this afternoon, and then Jeffrey came into the house holding his shoulder."

Trampoline? That contraption (and the skateboard) must have been invented by an orthopedist.

"Okay, let's take a look," I told her.

Jeffrey whimpered while I gently examined his shoulder and clavicle. There was a tender, swollen area over the midshaft of his collarbone, and a couple of X-rays defined the problem.

"He's broken his clavicle," I told her. "But he's going to be fine. Everything else looks good. He'll need an arm sling for a couple of weeks and some ice and Tylenol. Just try to keep him as quiet as possible—and off that trampoline—until this break has healed."

Jeffrey was five, and this was another of those greenstick fractures. The bone was bent but not separated. It was going to do great. Most clavicle fractures do until we reach our mid to late teens and beyond. Then the bone frequently breaks in two. That can sometimes happen with a younger child, but the treatment and outcome will usually be the same. An orthopedist once told me that with a complete fracture of a clavicle in a child Jeffrey's age, "All you have to do is get the two ends in the same room and it will heal great." Not so with a 19-year-old or older adult. These injuries are more complicated beyond childhood. They frequently require surgery to repair.

But not with Jeffrey or the majority of these fractures in our pediatric patients.

I hope you noticed the recommended treatment for this injury—a simple arm sling. A lot of parents think more needs to be done. After all, this is a fracture, isn't it? We used to do more—a figure-eight bandage that wrapped behind a child's neck and under his armpits. We would cinch this up as tight as possible, pulling those shoulders back as much as we could. But that was really painful for the child and completely unnecessary with more complications, pain, and frustration yet no difference in healing or any good outcome. In hindsight, it seems pretty barbaric. A simple arm sling works best. If you find yourself in an ER or clinic and someone tries to do anything more than that, pull out this book and open it to this chapter.

And you might ask the health care provider if he knows the difference between a fracture, a break, and a crack.

> *"As far as her mom was concerned, tea fixed everything.*
> *Have a cold? Have some tea.*
> *Broken bones? There's tea for that too.*
> *Somewhere in her mother's pantry, Laurel suspected,*
> *was a box of tea that said,*
> *'In case of Armageddon, steep three to five minutes.'"*

Aprilynne Pike

# ADHD—Diagnosis

## ✚ Everybody says my kid is hyper. Should we start him on some medication?

Whoa! Wait a minute. Wait a couple of minutes. You might be thinking that because your child is "hyper," he has ADHD and needs some form of treatment. That might be true, but let's be sure of what we're talking about. ADHD is a common cause of being "hyper," but not the only one. And because ADHD is so common, we need to know something about it.

Let's start with the name. ADHD stands for attention deficit hyperactivity disorder. That's the last time we're going to write it all out, but we need to keep every word in mind, because they define the condition.

ADHD has two components—*attention deficit* and *hyperactivity*. They both affect behavior, emotion, and thinking as well as academic performance and social functioning. And both have their own set of core symptoms. That's important to know, because those symptoms alert us to the presence of this disorder and also allow us to monitor their improvement through various forms of treatment. We're going to start with the *hyperactivity* part.

This is what we're most familiar with and most accustomed to seeing, either in our own child or in someone

> "Living with ADHD is like being locked in a room with 100 televisions and 100 radios all playing. None of them have power buttons so you can turn them off and the door is locked from the outside."
>
> **SARAH YOUNG**

else's. Hyperactivity almost always occurs with *impulsive* behavior and is usually seen by the time a child reaches four years of age. The symptoms will increase over the next three or four years and peak when the child reaches seven or eight. After that, the hyperactive symptoms begin to subside. By the teenage years, the hyperactivity might barely be noticeable, yet the adolescent can still have feelings of restlessness and be unable to settle down. The impulsive symptoms, on the other hand, frequently persist throughout life. That's a real problem for the untreated individual. In the wrong environment, this impulsivity can put a child at risk for alcohol abuse, the abuse of other substances, and involvement in what should be obviously dangerous activities. Even driving can become dangerous when the impulsivity leads to recklessness. (The majority of traffic accidents involving teenagers are caused by those with untreated ADHD.)

Here are some of the symptoms we see with hyperactivity and impulsivity:

- difficulty remaining seated at school or work
- fidgeting (squirming while seated, tapping feet or hands)
- acting or speaking without thinking (the child doesn't seem to have a "filter")
- difficulty playing quietly
- excessive talking
- in younger children, running around or climbing on any available object
- feelings of restlessness in adolescents
- blurting answers too quickly
- difficulty taking turns
- interrupting others when they're talking
- always on the go and difficult to keep up with[1]

Now for the *attention deficit* part of ADHD. This is usually referred to as "inattention," and it's marked by a reduced ability to focus attention and a reduced speed of thinking/cognitive processing, including correct responding. These children are described as sluggish thinkers, and they frequently appear to be daydreaming. Usually the complaints center on thought and academic problems. These symptoms typically are not apparent until the child is eight or nine years of age, when academic abilities begin to shake out. Like what we see with the impulsive component of this disorder, symptoms of inattention usually last a lifetime.

Before we go further, this is a good time to stress this important point: The impulsivity and inattentiveness of ADHD can last a lifetime. Many of us think this is a disorder experienced by only young children, maybe pushing into the teenage years. After that, they should "grow out of it." It doesn't work that way. Many adults go through life needlessly struggling with ADHD. Their work suffers, their relationships suffer, and their ability to parent suffers.

> "Be kind, for everyone you meet is fighting a hard battle."
>
> **PLATO**

So what are the core symptoms of this attention deficit? Here's what we see:

- difficulty maintaining attention in school, at play, and in the home
- the inability to pay close attention to detail and making careless mistakes
- failure to follow through with chores at home or with homework
- the inability to follow a two- or three-step direction: "Go to your room, pick up your dirty clothes, and brush your teeth."
- appearing not to listen, even when being directly addressed
- avoiding tasks that will require consistent and focused mental effort

- losing objects/tools needed for specific tasks and activities (schoolbooks, musical instruments, sports equipment)

- forgetfulness in routine activities, such as homework and assigned household chores

- difficulty organizing tasks, activities, and personal belongings

- easily distracted by things that are unimportant and inconsequential

With these core symptoms in mind, we can begin to determine if our child might have a problem with ADHD. To meet this diagnosis, we need evidence of impaired functioning—significant problems with academic and social activities. Here's how the American Psychiatric Association (APA) currently defines criteria for the diagnosis of ADHD:

For children 17 and younger, there must be six or more symptoms of hyperactivity and impulsivity or six or more symptoms of inattention. (For adults, that number is only five symptoms.) In addition, these symptoms must

- occur often

- be present in more than one setting, such as both school and home

- persist for at least six months

- be present *before* age 12

- significantly impair function in academic and social activities

- be excessive for the developmental level of the child[2]

✚ *I think my child has just about all of these! Does that mean he has both the hyperactive and attention deficit type of ADHD?*

That's possible. Let's take a moment to work through this. Let's say your child has six of the core symptoms of hyperactivity/impulsivity but only three of those listed under attention deficit. That would satisfy the APA's criteria for ADHD of the hyperactive subtype (there are three subtypes, this being one of them). On the other hand, if only three of the hyperactive/impulsivity core symptoms are present but six of the attention deficit core symptoms, this still qualifies as ADHD of the inattentive subtype. If you're right about your child, and he has six or more core symptoms in each group, he would fall into the subtype of having a *combined* ADHD disorder. This subtyping is important because it will guide appropriate treatment, help set reasonable and achievable goals, and give a framework for monitoring your child's progress.

> "ADHD has a strong genetic predisposition. Up to 80 percent of children with ADHD have a parent with the same diagnosis."[3]

If these criteria are met, validated screening tools can firmly establish a diagnosis of ADHD. While you can find some of these tools online, if you think your child has many of these symptoms, you'll be better served by asking your pediatrician or family physician to provide further guidance. These validated screening tools should be completed by as many current and past schoolteachers of your child as possible, along with anyone who has worked closely with her or knows her well. The more people and opinions involved here, the more help your physician will have in making a correct assessment.

The important point is to first think through all this and know your child. Then if you think he needs help, get it. Untreated, the negative consequences of ADHD are poor academic performance with limited future opportunities, poor social functioning, peer rejection, poor self-esteem, increased risk for depression and anxiety—and for your teenager, greater risk taking. With the correct diagnosis, the treatment can be straightforward and effective.

But getting back to your question...If someone thinks your child is hyper, don't take offense. Take notice. This issue is not about you;

it's about your child. There's no room here for anyone but your child, and there's absolutely no room for denial. Make no mistake, your child's happiness and well-being may depend on a proper diagnosis and treatment.

*"ADHD is not a choice or bad parenting.*
*Kids with ADHD work twice as hard as their peers every day*
*but receive more negative feedback from the world."*

Author Unknown

# 15

# ADHD—Treatment

### ✤ What's the best way to treat ADHD?

First, we need to understand that ADHD is a *chronic* disorder. It's not like tonsillitis, where an effective antibiotic will take care of the problem, or like a greenstick fracture in the wrist that will heal in four to six weeks. This is a problem that's going to stay with your child—maybe for life. We hope the symptoms will improve as they get older, but we also need to look at ADHD with a long view. The good news is that if treated appropriately, the symptoms of ADHD can be controlled and long-term prospects and potential are greatly enhanced.

Now for the steps of treatment.

Because this is a chronic and complicated condition, the best approach is through a team. This will of course involve engaged parents but also other family members and schoolteachers. We need to stress the importance of regular communication with your child's teacher, and we'll look at ways to effectively do that a little later. The team includes your pediatrician/family physician, perhaps a counselor, and maybe even a dietician.

> "ADHD—It's like being a cat with 100 people with laser pointers."
>
> **JAMIE HYNDS**

The importance of family involvement needs to be stressed as well. Your child (depending on their age), their siblings (depending on their ages), and you as parents need to talk about the issue, understand it as much as possible, and discuss various treatment options and goals. Setting those target goals, especially academic and behavioral, has to be a joint decision, and the goals have to be reasonable and manageable.

Those goals should be limited, with three to no more than six outcomes addressed at any one time. These target goals might include the following:

- improved relationships with siblings, teachers, and parents
- improved academic performance
- improvement in following rules at both home and school

Academic performance can be assessed with the regular reporting of grades, but these other areas can be graded with a report card as well, designed by the team and used daily. This is where you want your child's teacher involved and willing to help. And just so you know, your pediatrician or treating clinician will want your input into changed behavior and performance, but they'll certainly want (and probably value more) the opinion of your child's teacher. No offense, but their views will be more objective and dispassionate.

> "I wish I could sleep but my ADHD kicks in and...
> one sheep, two sheep, cow, turtle, duck, old McDonald had a farm...
> hey Macarena!"
>
> **AUTHOR UNKNOWN**

As we begin our treatment plan, we also need to search for the existence of coexisting conditions—things that could be making the ADHD worse or even causing the symptoms instead of ADHD itself. As many as one-third of children with ADHD might have one or more coexisting conditions, including mood disorders, anxiety, opposition defiant disorder, learning disabilities, tics, and sleep disorders. We need to stress the importance of considering the presence of a sleep problem, evaluating it, and then getting treatment if needed. One thing is for certain—treating a coexisting sleep disorder will greatly improve the chances of successfully treating ADHD.

We have a variety of treatment strategies available to us, and the initial choice will usually depend on the age of the child. For instance, most experts agree that preschool children (ages four to five) should begin with behavior therapy rather than medication. These behavioral interventions include modifications in the child's physical and social environment. These will, hopefully, change behavior by using rewards and nonpunitive consequences. Some of these include positive reinforcement, time-outs, the use of a "token economy" (receiving small tokens for proper behaviors and responses that can be exchanged for specified items or activities), and response cost (lost privileges or rewards withheld when problem behavior occurs).

This seems like a lot, and it is. We're going to provide you with references that will give you much more information and help you with the best behavioral and other strategies for your child, but here are some things you can do right now:

- Develop and maintain a consistent daily schedule.

- Keep unnecessary distractions to a minimum.

- Provide easily accessible, specific, and logical places for your child to keep schoolwork, toys, and clothes.

- Reward positive behavior. You might want to look into the token economy idea.

- Set small, understandable, and achievable goals.

- Use charts and checklists to help your child stay "on task."

- Limit choices—activities, food, almost everything.

- Find activities your child enjoys and can be successful doing. We all need a passion—maybe a couple of them.

- Examine your own behavior and identify any unintentional reinforcement on your part that might be creating negative behaviors.

- Make sure your discipline is calm (time-outs, removing your child from an aggravating situation, providing constructive distraction).

That said, this is a great place to remind ourselves of what the apostle Paul tells us in his letter to the Galatians. In chapter 5, verses 22 through 23, he lists the "fruit of the Spirit." These are virtues that God's

Holy Spirit produces in the lives and hearts of believers. Thankfully, it's the work of the Spirit that does this, because none of us has the inherent capability. Here are the nine fruits:

- love
- joy
- peace
- forbearance (patience)
- kindness
- goodness
- faithfulness
- gentleness
- self-control

Isn't this what we all need? And isn't each of these crucial to how we approach our child with ADHD? We need to consider each fruit one by one and examine our own hearts.

While we're still talking about preschool children, we need to consider those circumstances where medication might be added to behavioral strategies. Some examples of those circumstances might be:

- your child posing a significant risk of injury to other children or caregivers
- expulsion (or threatened expulsion) from preschool or day care
- suspected or documented central nervous system injury (some of these could be prenatal, such as alcohol or cocaine exposure) and prematurity—less than 32 weeks gestation
- the existence of a strong family history of ADHD
- the symptoms of ADHD remaining uncontrolled and interfering with other therapies

With school-aged children (older than six) and adolescents, initial management is probably going to include stimulant medication along with behavioral therapy. Parental and family preferences will weigh heavily here, and they need to be thoroughly discussed.

As we've noted several times, ADHD is a chronic disease that needs to be monitored regularly, looking for the response to therapy, for adverse reactions to medications (if given), and for adherence to the treatment plan. If we fail to see a satisfactory response, the two most likely causes are not adhering to the plan or our failing to identify one of the coexisting problems noted earlier. At that point, we should call a time-out and reevaluate.

The frequency of follow-up visits depends on several factors, including the age of the child, whether or not she is receiving medication, and how well the core symptoms and target behaviors are being controlled. Visits might be once or twice a year, monthly, or even more frequent, especially during the initial stages of treatment. Every child needs an individualized plan.

Measuring the response to treatment can be done through teacher interviews and reports, use of the daily report cards we previously discussed, and reviewing academic performance. Improvement isn't going to happen overnight, but we hope to see a positive response over the first few weeks of treatment.

### ✚ What about other stuff, like elimination diets and chelation? Do they work?

If you search the internet, you'll find lots of things that promise improvement for ADHD—perhaps even a cure. Beware. Most of these are unproven and potentially dangerous. Let's consider the ones you mentioned.

Elimination diets haven't been proven to be of benefit, and the influence of diet on hyperactivity, attention, and behavior is controversial. One exception could be caffeine. It's a stimulant, and it might help your child a little. But it's easy for children to consume too much of it, creating a negative effect on their behavior and attention. We recommend avoiding it as much as possible.

Dietary factors such as food additives, food intolerance, or food allergy usually don't affect behavior and aren't significant in the majority of ADHD cases. But if you believe something your child is eating or drinking is making him worse, eliminate it and see what happens. Eliminate one thing at a time, though, so you're making a correct identification. You don't want to overcomplicate your or your child's life. It's complicated enough already. (Essential fatty acid supplementation has been recommended, but no concrete evidence exists to support its use. It won't be harmful, but you can save your money.)

Stay away from "chelation therapy" and megavitamins; they have the potential for serious side effects. They, along with other complementary and alternative medicines such as herbal and mineral supplements, St. John's wort, and several forms of visual training, haven't been proven helpful. Stick with what we know works and is safe.

The more you know about ADHD, the better you'll be able to help your child. Here is a list of useful resources. There's a lot of information here; however, the better we understand this problem, the less intimidating it will seem.

- Attention Deficit Disorder Association (ADDA)—www. add.org
- The American Academy of Child and Adolescent Psychiatry (AACAP)— www.aacap.org
- Children and Adults with Attention Deficit/Hyperactivity Disorder (CHADD)—www.chadd.org
- National Institute of Mental Health—www.nimh.nih.gov/ health/publications/adhd-listing.shtml
- American Academy of Pediatrics—aap.org

> *"Forgive your child and yourself nightly. You didn't ask to live with the effects of ADHD any more than did your child."*
>
> Martin L. Kutscher

# 16

# ADHD—Medications

### ✛ What's the best ADHD medication for my child?

This is a situation where one size doesn't fit all, and we have to fight the temptation to think it does.

When we think about medication for ADHD, most of us probably immediately think of an amphetamine—particularly Adderall. While that drug might be indicated for your child, many factors should go into making that choice. Not taking the time to consider these factors can result in treatment failure, adverse reactions, and compounded frustration. Let's look at how we should go about making the important decision of whether to start a medication, which one it should be, and at what dose.

Before any prescription is written, your physician should gather a detailed patient and family history regarding the presence of any cardiovascular disease. A focused cardiovascular physical exam should follow, along with your child's baseline height, weight, blood pressure, and heart rate. This is important because the stimulants used with ADHD can cause an increase in blood pressure and heart rate. A doctor wants to be sure medication isn't going to cause an unnecessary complication.

> "Living with ADHD is like walking up a down escalator. You can get there eventually, but the journey is exhausting."
>
> **KATHLEEN ELY**

In addition, the presence of potential medication side effects should be explored *before* any medicine is started. It will be important to know which is the cart and which is the horse should any of these reactions occur. These include, among other things, sleep disturbances, abdominal pain, moodiness, changes in appetite, headaches, and tics. (Tics are sudden, repetitive movements or involuntary sounds, such as eye blinking, shoulder shrugging, facial grimacing, or throat clearing. They can sometimes be a side effect of ADHD medications, but more often the medications are unmasking a preexisting problem. That's why it's important to explore these things ahead of time.) If your child is an adolescent, there should be a thorough assessment for any existing or potential for substance use or abuse.

Once we've done these things, it's important to make sure you and your child (if age appropriate) understand the purpose of treatment with medications, how they work, what problems to look for, and what to expect. If there is no history of appetite problems, tics, or sleeping disorders, these specifically need to be discussed as possibilities and addressed should they arise. This is the time to ask questions—a lot of them. Make sure you get the answers you need.

When the decision to start medication is made, understand that it will usually take from one to three months to determine the best medication, dosage, and frequency of administration for your child. Keeping that in mind will help avoid frustration during this adjustment/ finding the right dose, especially with the need for frequent follow-ups—maybe weekly for a while.

Remember, one size doesn't fit all, and to help drive home that point, here are some things to consider before selecting a medication:

- the duration of the desired medication coverage (Short-acting stimulants last about four hours, but what are we trying to cover? Is that enough time? Does the window need to be extended to midafternoon or early evening?)

- the time of day the child's target symptoms are the worst

- whether the child can swallow pills or capsules

- whether the medication could/should be given at school

- whether there are preexisting problems, such as tics or headaches

- the potential side effects of a particular medication
- whether the child has a history/potential for substance abuse or someone in the home has that potential
- the cost of the drug (In general, short-acting stimulants are much less expensive than the longer acting ones, and generics are less expensive than brand names. And while generics work just as well as brand names, they're not always available in the same dosages, making their use more problematic at times.)

While there are several classes of medications to choose from, most experts will recommend the use of a stimulant, including amphetamines (Ritalin, Adderall), methylphenidate (Metadate), or lisdexamfetamine (Vyvanse). Choosing to use a stimulant is based on a rapid onset of action and a long track record of safety and success. Other classes of drugs can be employed as well, including *alpha adrenergics* (Tenex and clonidine), which are useful in young children (ages five to six), especially if anger issues are present. We're going to limit our discussion of ADHD medications to the use of stimulants.

Let's start with the rapid/short-acting forms. These should be the initial choice in children under six years of age, mainly because children that age are more sensitive to higher doses of these medicines and longer-acting preparations don't come in the smaller doses they require. Effects from the medicine can be seen within as little as 30 minutes, with a peak effect between two or three hours. This is important to know since timing is everything here. This is another question to ask your physician and to keep in mind as you monitor your child's day and needs.

Intermediate or long-acting drugs are generally used with children

> "It's like opening 100 tabs in your browser at once and trying to do something different in each one at the same time. Then someone walks up and wants to have a conversation."
>
> **JENNIFER ARNOTT**

who require a duration of action longer than four hours or with whom giving medicine every four hours poses a problem. They make it easier to be sure your child gets the coverage she needs and improve adherence to the treatment plan. Another advantage is that they're less likely to be abused because they don't have the immediate "pop" of the short-acting forms. They're more expensive, though, so you need to keep that in mind. As a rule, you won't see an effect for a couple of hours, and it will be more gradual than the rapid-acting forms, with the peak happening around seven hours.

It's perfectly acceptable—maybe preferable—to combine a long-acting drug in the morning with a short-acting one in the afternoon to give extended coverage when needed. Again, this all depends on your child, the setting, and his needs.

In the beginning, it's all about finding the right medicine and the right dose, with the goal of reaching our target with minimal or no side effects. Here are some points to keep in mind:

- These drugs are not weight based (such as an antibiotic for a five-year-old), because every child's metabolism is different and the way they handle these medications differs.

- It's helpful to start these medicines on a weekend so you'll be able to observe the initial response and watch for any side effects.

- All of these stimulant medications should be started at the lowest possible dose and increased gradually as needed (usually every three to seven days). We want to see an improvement in the core symptoms of about 50 percent (without the development of side effects), and this can be apparent in as little as 30 to 40 minutes after the drug is given.

- High-fat meals can delay the onset of some of these drugs and even increase the peak concentrations.

- If the drug needs to be stopped, it's perfectly safe to do so at once—cold turkey. There's no need to gradually taper this medication.

### ✚ What are the side effects we should be looking for?

These are powerful medications, and while effective and safe, they can produce some unwanted reactions:

- *Decreased appetite and weight loss.* This is by far the most common side effect. If this happens, it's not a reason to stop the medication. Try giving it at or after a meal, and make sure your child has access to calorie-dense but nutritious foods.

- *The potential for poor growth.* A "drug holiday" might be tried if this happens, but it should be based on a series of measurements and the use of growth charts. Your physician can help with that.

- *Sleep disorders.* This might come in the form of nightmares and insomnia. The best initial approach is to ensure your child has a good sleep routine and environment (dark, cool, quiet).

- *Dizziness.* This is rare. Make sure your child is getting plenty of fluids, and during one of these episodes, take her pulse and write it down.

- *Tics.* Also rare. We mentioned these earlier, and if they should start or worsen while on the medication, the dose may need to be lowered or stopped altogether.

- *Rebound.* This occurs as the medication is wearing off in the afternoon or evening and usually lasts 30 to 60 minutes. The problem symptoms return and may even be worse. Here's where a longer-acting form can be used or we can add a rapid/short-acting medicine to cover the problem time period.

- *Moodiness.* This, in addition to increased activity, sadness, or irritability, is common with short-acting drugs as they wear off. Again, a longer-acting form or adding a short-acting one in the evening might help.

- *Headaches.* If the medication causes headaches, they'll usually occur within one to two hours of taking it. If headaches become a daily problem, patients can try a different stimulant.

This all sounds complicated, but with the understanding of a few key points—peak effects, coverage, combining short- and long-acting drugs—there should be a successful medication regimen for your child. And if one stimulant doesn't give you the desired response, at least 50 percent of the time a different one will. The same is true with side effects. You might see the development of a tic or insomnia with one drug but not with another. Don't give up, but learn all you can. And make sure your physician is experienced in the treatment of ADHD and is aware of these concerns and options. A good idea is to go to your child's first visit with a list of the behaviors you want to see addressed, the problems your child is having at home and at school, and the times of day and week when they're the most difficult.

Now the good news: If your child has been correctly diagnosed as having ADHD and the correct medication/dosing/timing has been selected, the response rate to this treatment is about 70 percent—and even higher, according to some studies. That's a huge number and cause for optimism and hope. This not only includes improvement in the core symptoms of ADHD but also in the relationship between you and your child. That's what we're trying to accomplish, isn't it? But it has to be done thoughtfully, carefully, and with patience.

> *"I know what it's like to grow up with ADHD*
> *and how important it is for parents, caregivers and patients*
> *to have access to accurate information."*
>
> Ty Pennington

# 17

# Hearing Loss

*+ Our babysitter thinks our 18-month-old son can't hear. We've started paying more attention, and now we think she might be right. How do we check that out?*

Hearing loss is the number one impairment in older adults. Almost always, its onset is gradual, frequently starting in the teenage and young adult years. It's—

"What?"

We said *hearing loss*...Oh, never mind. Just remember that much of our hearing loss is noise induced—noise that's too loud and for too long a time. The threshold for the amount of noise that causes damage is different for each of us, so we need to be careful early on. Those ear-buds and headsets delivering damaging decibels to teenagers' eardrums will take their toll. It starts with knocking out their ability to hear high frequencies, and it doesn't come back. Not only do you need to know *what* your children are listening to; you need to know *how loud* it is.

But you were asking about your 18-month-old son and whether he might have a hearing deficit. We need to start by asking questions about your family history, any problems during your pregnancy, any medical conditions your child has had...a bunch of stuff. But let's tell you how this usually presents.

> Sally is a two-year-old who has been in good health. Her mother brings her in because "She's just not talking right." There's been no history of any medical problems or family history of a hearing problem. When asked about the new-born hearing screen she had in the hospital, her mother

answers that it wasn't "quite right," and they were told to have it repeated at some time in the future. She thought her daughter seemed fine until now, and that recommendation had "just slipped" her mind. After preliminary testing and an evaluation by an audiologist, Sally is now wearing hearing aids because of her moderate bilateral hearing loss.

And then there's this:

Billy, a five-year-old boy, is brought to the clinic by his mother for his first-ever visit. She paces the room with arms folded across her chest, shaking her head. "Billy needs some medicine for ADHD. Everybody thinks so. He won't pay attention, and he's all over the place. He's starting to have trouble in preschool, and his teachers want us to do something." A glance through the records she brings reveals that Billy has had multiple episodes of ear infections—not enough to warrant an ENT referral but more than normal. An exam of his ears reveals scarring and retraction of his eardrums, with fluid in both middle ears. After the insertion of tubes by an ENT specialist, he's no longer "all over the place" and is doing great in school. And he's not taking any ADHD medication.

Hearing loss in young children can be subtle and difficult to pick up. In fact, that's the rule rather than the exception. It's common, affecting about 3 to 4 per 1,000 newborns. It's important to catch hearing problems, because early identification and treatment for these infants can improve their chances of keeping up with their unimpaired peers. No detection and treatment can lead to delayed language development, difficulty with behavior, and poor cognitive and academic performance. That's going to be true for whenever the hearing loss develops, whether it's congenital or, as in Billy's case, it develops over the first few years of life. Those years—the first 36 months—are crucial when it comes to language and cognitive development.

Sally's mother mentioned her daughter's newborn hearing test. How in the world do you check a newborn's hearing? First, every state in the

US requires a hearing screen be done before a newborn leaves the hospital. The procedure itself is quick and relatively easy. A newborn isn't going to respond to a voice or other noise in a meaningful or predictable way, so the person doing the test inserts a small microphone into the ear canal and measures the sounds that come back from the inner ear. The newborns don't have to do anything; they just lie there. A normal test doesn't mean everything is necessarily fine, only that you can wait a while before more formal testing. If it's abnormal (like with Sally), the child will need more testing sooner, preferably within three months.

These risk factors for hearing loss in a newborn should be red flags:

- specific in-utero infections (mainly viruses)
- genetic disorders (about 400 of these exist)
- a family history of hearing deficits
- ear and other facial abnormalities noted at birth
- a significantly elevated bilirubin level during the first few days of life
- low birth weight
- a low Apgar score at birth—3 or less at five minutes
- five or more days spent in the Neonatal Intensive Care Unit (NICU)
- exposure to several specific antibiotics known to damage the hearing mechanism

Beyond the newborn period is a different set of red flags for hearing loss.

- frequent middle-ear infections (*otitis media*)—the most common cause
- trauma
- foreign bodies (ears are a kid's favorite repository for beans, beads, and anything else that will fit in her ear canal)

- genetic syndromes that were unknown and undiagnosed at birth but are manifest at one or two years of age

✚ *That's a lot to think about! What are some simple things we should be looking for with our child?*

Here's a simple "hearing checklist" for your infant or toddler:

- Birth to 3 months

  ○ Your child becomes quiet around usual and everyday voices and noises.

  ○ He reacts to loud sounds by blinking, waking up, or startled movements.

  ○ She makes soft baby gurgles while awake.

- 3 to 6 months

  ○ Your child will turn his head and eyes toward normal sounds, such as voices, a barking dog, or the beeping fire truck Uncle Robbie gave him.

  ○ She starts to make simple sounds like "ba," "ooh," and "ga."

  ○ You'll notice a reaction when you change the tone of your voice.

- 6 to 9 months

  ○ Your child now responds to soft sounds, such as talking.

  ○ He begins to respond to his own name.

  ○ She understands simple words such as "bye-bye" and "no."

- 9 to 12 months

  ○ Your child will repeat single words and begin to copy animal sounds.

- When asked, he will point to favorite toys or food.

- She consistently responds to soft and loud noises.

- 12 to 18 months

  - Your child will follow simple spoken instructions, such as "Pick up the spoon" or "Get the ball."

  - You'll notice him bouncing to music.

  - She's using ten or more words.

  - When asked, he will point to specific people, body parts, or toys.

- 18 to 24 months

  - Your child is now using 20 or more words.

  - She listens to simple stories or songs.

  - He's now able to combine two or more words, such as "more juice."

- 2 to 3 years

  - Your child can follow two-step instructions, like "Pick up the block and put it in the box."

  - She's using sentences with two or three words.

  - At age two, his speech is understood *some* of the time—maybe as much as 50 percent.

  - By age three, you should be able to understand most of her speech—at least 75 percent of the time.

If your child is a little older and can communicate with you, pay attention to the following:

- Your child frequently asks, "What?" and seems to be doing it more often. (This is normal and acceptable behavior in husbands, but it can be a sign of hearing loss in your child.)

- When watching the TV, your child turns up the volume louder than other members of the family do.

- When talking with you, she focuses on your face, especially your mouth.

- He turns his head when listening and might even mention "That's my good ear."

- She doesn't seem to pay attention.

- His hearing seems fine some of the time and not so good at others.

- She's beginning to experience problems in school, and her teacher, if astute, might bring a potential hearing problem to your attention.

- He begins to speak more loudly—an early tip-off.

If you notice any of these things, or if you just have a gut feeling, it's time to have your child examined. As we noted earlier, the sooner hearing loss is addressed, the better off your child is going to be.

The American Academy of Pediatrics has established some guidelines for hearing screening. They recommend that all children be tested at the ages of four, five, six, eight, and ten. After ten, the guideline calls for testing once between 11 and 14, once between 15 and 17, and once between 18 and 21. That seems like a lot of testing, but it's the only way to diagnose a hearing problem before it causes significant complications or becomes permanent.

We want our child's first word to be "Mama" or "Papa," not "What?"

> *"When someone in the family has a hearing loss,*
> *the entire family has a hearing problem."*

Mark Ross

# 18

# Seat Belts and Car Seats

### ✚ At what age is it okay for our child to ride in the backseat without a seat belt?

Seriously? We're physicians, and a couple of things make us cringe as we drive down the highway or maneuver through the streets of our city. The first is to pull up beside someone in a closed-up car and watch as the driver puffs on a cigarette, exhales a cloud of carcinogens into their vehicle, and then turns to say something to a two-year-old in the backseat. *What are they thinking?* The answer has to be that they're not. It's one thing to make the decision to pollute your own lungs, but your child's? That's a hard thing to see and disturbingly cringeworthy.

The other thing is even worse. Much worse. One of us witnessed an example of this just a few days ago.

It was a Monday morning, a little before eight o'clock, and I was on my way to the clinic. I was driving behind a small sedan, trying to keep a safe distance behind the female driver. That wasn't easy as she unpredictably slowed down and then sped up—over and over—on the two-lane country road. The road was too twisting to try to pass her, so I resigned myself to being cautious and exercising as much patience as I could muster.

During one of those slow-down spells, I noticed the toddler in the backseat. At first I couldn't be sure, but when the little boy moved from one side of the car to the other, I knew. He wasn't in a car seat or even in a seat belt. He was unrestrained—a disaster waiting to happen. My patience evaporated, and I wondered what I could do to protect him.

I glanced beyond the sedan, knowing we were approaching a stop sign. The driver must have been unfamiliar with the road and didn't expect the upcoming intersection. Almost too late, she slammed on her brakes, swerved from side to side, and came to a sudden stop a few feet from the sign. I hadn't been watching the car, just the boy in the backseat. He had been standing in the middle of the car when she slammed on the brakes, and he was violently thrown forward. He bounced off the back of the woman's seat and then caromed toward the front passenger side. His arms went out, and he somehow grabbed the passenger headrest, held on for dear life, and managed to avoid going through the windshield.

The driver looked in the rearview mirror, caught my eye, and shook her head. Then she looked down at the boy. He was wide-eyed and seemed about to burst into tears, but he was apparently unhurt. She started laughing, and I watched as he gave her a nervous smile and they drove away.

That was a near miss. I looked down and realized I was white-knuckling my steering wheel. It wasn't out of fear for my own safety; it was the memory of something that had happened a few years earlier.

*Seven thirty p.m.*

The crew from EMS 2 had just rolled their stretcher into the ER, carrying a young man who didn't appear to be in any distress.

"Auto accident at the intersection of Mt. Gallant and Celanese," the paramedic told me. He tilted his head to the young man and added, "Just a few scratches and a sore shoulder, nothing bad."

His partner pulled me aside and spoke quietly. "EMS 1 is bringing the woman from the other vehicle. She's okay, too, but her little boy..." He paused, looked at the floor, and shook his head. "He's not okay. It's going to be tough."

Two highway patrolmen approached the nurses' station and dropped their notebooks on the countertop. They told me what happened.

The young man EMS 2 brought in was an 18-year-old college student. He had been traveling west on Celanese Road and had a green light through the busy Mt. Gallant intersection. Heading into the intersection on Mt. Gallant was a young mother driving a late-model SUV. For whatever reason, she didn't see the red light and barreled through the crossroads. The college student slammed on his brakes but couldn't help T-boning the SUV, causing it to spin 360 degrees before flipping and landing on its side. The young woman was gripping the steering wheel—wild-eyed and screaming. But she was safe—restrained by her seat belt and shoulder harness.

Her three-year-old son had been sipping a Coke, sitting in the middle of the backseat, unbelted and unrestrained. At impact, he was thrown against the back-left door, breaking his left upper arm. As the van spun violently, he was thrown across the backseat and into the passenger-side window. The force with which he struck the glass was enough to break it and his neck. When the SUV flipped over, he was ejected from the vehicle and landed 15 feet away in the middle of the intersection. The first responders found him in a pool of blood—no pulse and no respirations. His mother screamed in the background.

As the patrolman finished telling me this story, the ambulance doors opened. EMS 1 silently pushed their stretcher past the nurses' station and down the hallway.

*"If only. Those must be the two saddest words in the world."*

Mercedes Lackey

# 19

# Lumps and Bumps

✦ *We noticed this knot on our boy's chest
a couple of days ago. What do you think it is?*

You might be surprised how often this concern brings a parent and child to the office or sometimes to the ER. A mother or father discovers something unusual on their child and immediately starts to worry. That's understandable, and sometimes that something needs to be looked at.

Here are some things to be concerned about if you find a new growth or knot on your son or daughter.

- *The presence of fever.* Fever might indicate infection or significant inflammation.

- *Trauma.* Minor contusions and falls might be the cause of a subtle fracture, especially in young children and infants.

- *Tenderness localized over a "long bone"—the arms or legs.* While rare, this tenderness might be how a bone cancer initially presents.

- *Swelling, redness, tenderness anywhere.* These symptoms could be the start of an abscess.

- *Swollen and tender knots under the neck, in the armpits, or in the groin.* Some kind of lymph node pathology might be getting started.

- *Any prolonged illness (weeks or months), with fatigue and weight loss.* When this happens, we have to start looking for a cause.

- *Unusual skin rashes.* A rash could be infection, but it could also be something coming from the bone marrow.

We'll want to know about timing. When did this symptom start? In your case, you found this knot a couple of days ago, but in the majority of circumstances, what a parent is seeing or feeling has been there for a while—weeks or months or even years. That's true with children and especially true with adults. We rub our heads, scratch our backs, look in the mirror, and there it is—something we never noticed before. We need to be careful yet use common sense.

A few specific concerns frequently bring parents into the office, and we want you to be aware of them.

*The Xiphoid Process.* Pronounced "zif-oid," the xiphoid is the boney lower end of the sternum. By process, we mean it starts out as cartilage but gradually calcifies during childhood. The root word is from the Greek and means "sword-like." If you Google "xiphoid," you'll see why. It's pointy, like a sword. The Latin root for this word must be "Don't keep rubbing it or it's going to become inflamed, swollen, and tender." That's usually when we see it with teenagers or adults. They find it one day, start rubbing it, and it becomes aggravated. But this is normal anatomy, and like most normal anatomy, there are a lot of normal variations. The xiphoid can be short, long, curved inward, or even curved outward. It's never going to be a problem if you keep your hands off it.

*The Greater Occipital Tuberosity (Protuberance).* Sounds like one of the titles for the wizard in the kingdom of Oz, doesn't it? The occipital protuberance is normal anatomy as well, and it's the knot you feel at the base of your skull. (Go ahead; try finding it.) It's there so the trapezius muscles—as well as one of the strong ligaments in the back of the neck—have something to attach to. It varies in size, and when it's a little large, its discovery can cause alarm. Relax. It's been there all your life or all your child's life. Once again, it's never going to cause a problem.

*A Swollen and Tender Front of the Knee—Osgood-Schlatter Disease.* Named after an American and a Swiss physician, this is a common problem, usually seen in children between the ages of 9 and 14. It's related to physical activity or playing sports, and historically it's been more common on boys. However, with the growing participation of girls in athletics of all kinds, this distribution is evening out.

It's not really the knee that's involved but the boney protuberance just below the knee—the tibial (the big bone in the lower leg) tuberosity. (Go on; check this out too.) It's that big bump just below your kneecap. Part of the patellar tendon attaches here, and with repetitive contraction of the powerful quadriceps muscles and straightening of the knee, the immature growth plate in that area can partially separate, causing pain and swelling.

We typically see this in a 13- or 14-year-old boy or an 11- or 12-year-old girl (girls' muscles and bones mature earlier) and almost always after a gradual onset of symptoms. Mild pain, swelling, and a slight limp become worse with jumping, running, squatting, or climbing stairs. Rest makes it better. It's usually on one leg, though both legs can be affected at the same time. The diagnosis is made "clinically," meaning X-rays aren't needed. Exceptions would be those children whose pain occurs at night, who have sudden onset of pain or fever, or who have pain that's not over the tuberosity.

The treatment is conservative but effective with icing and acetaminophen or ibuprofen (for not more than a week). A knee pad might help as well. This doesn't start overnight, and it's not going away overnight—the usual course of resolution is from 6 to 18 months, with the symptoms coming and going. Restricted causative activities (such as those listed above) will speed the healing. There might be some residual and long-term swelling, depending on the extent of the separation and the length of time before addressing the problem, but it's benign and will go away.

So the majority of lumps and bumps and knots we find on our children are okay. Use common sense. If any of the red flags listed are present, get what you've found checked out. In the meantime, stop rubbing that knot on your boy's chest!

*"There are more things to alarm us than to harm us,*
*and we suffer more in apprehension than in reality."*

Seneca the Younger

# 20

# Lacerations

## + How do I know if my child needs stitches?

It depends. Not every cut requires sutures, and if we jump the gun and rush to the ER, we might end up spending a lot of time and money in exchange for a simple Band-Aid. On the other hand (or knee or face), if we neglect a significant wound, we run the risk of infection and unnecessary scarring. So here are some things to keep in mind when your child falls on the sidewalk or runs into one corner of a piece of furniture.

Lacerations that won't stop bleeding need to be checked. Direct pressure over a wound, maybe with some ice, will stop most bleeding within five minutes. Use a clock. Don't assume you can accurately estimate the passage of five minutes, especially when screaming or blood or both are involved. If the bleeding doesn't stop, someone needs to have a look.

If you see "white stuff" in the wound, the cut is most likely through the full thickness of the skin, and you're looking at fatty tissue. No big deal, but this wound will need thorough cleansing and some kind of closure.

A laceration over a joint—elbow, finger, knee—also needs attention. There will be a lot of tension on the wound, which increases the risk of it repeatedly popping open. These lacerations take a while to heal.

Don't take a chance with your child's face unless you're dealing with a minuscule puncture wound or a superficial scratch. While keeping in mind that it's impossible for the face to be cut without a scar as a result, we want the smallest scar possible. Often, this will require some kind of closure.

Let's consider the types of closure available. The goal is to "approximate" the wound edges, bringing them together without too much tension, so they can knit together. We can use synthetic sutures, skin glue (Dermabond), staples, and Steri-Strips. Each of these are appropriate in the right setting. The key is to understand the setting.

### ✚ But I don't want my child to have stitches. Just use some skin glue.

We wish it were that simple and painless. Skin glue has its uses but only with wounds that are superficial and not gaping. A good rule of thumb is that what you see is what you get. The width of a wound in its initial state will be close to the width of the final scar months and years later. That's why we want to approximate the wound as soon as we can. Here's another rule of thumb: At one week of healing, scar tissue is forming in the wound but it's weak. It takes at least six months for the scar to achieve its near final strength. And contrary to popular belief, a scar will never be as strong as the original, healthy skin.

So what about Steri-Strips? We should use these only to provide additional support in holding a wound together, never as a primary closure. The strips can also be useful once stitches have been removed, but they will stay in place for only a couple of days. Yet even that may be helpful and should be considered.

And, finally, when should we consider skin staples? The answer is not often. Accurate placement of staples requires proper training and experience, which apparently aren't common. They can be used successfully on the scalp, but their placement in other areas can lead to unnecessary scarring and a "step-off" between the wound edges. The sad truth is that staples in the acute setting (i.e., the ER) are frequently used as an expedient—they're quicker to use than well-placed sutures. And absent the hands of an experienced provider, the outcome will be much less satisfactory. This is one of those times when we need to speak up and ask about other options.

## ✚ Okay, so we have stitches.
## When can little Stevie take a bath?

Another good question. Most closed wounds will seal over in about 24 hours. After that time, it's safe to let the wound get wet but then quickly and gently dried. This is no license for an hour of soaking in the tub, but a shower should be fine. Again, pat the stitched wound dry right away and apply some kind of ointment. We don't need anything magical here, just triple antibiotic or Bacitracin.

What *might* be magical is what we use after the stitches come out. The general guideline is to remove stitches in the face in five to seven days and stitches everywhere else in ten to fourteen days. Sutures left longer than that will dig into the skin and cause scarring themselves. (We've seen them still in place for as long as three or four months!)

Now the magic. We want to heal the wound and minimize scarring, so we advise parents to apply Vaseline once the sutures are removed. That's right, apply simple, old-fashioned Vaseline to the wound twice a day for a week or two. A thin film is all you need, and the results are as good or better than the much higher priced "scar reducers" you can find online and at your drugstore or even get by prescription. And if the wound is in a sun-exposed area of the skin, we recommend use of sunscreen (at least 50 SPF) for a few months.

Lacerations are going to happen, so be prepared—and try not to panic.

> *"How poor are they that have not patience!*
> *What wound did ever heal but by degrees?"*
>
> William Shakespeare

# 21

# Limps

**✛ *Our six-year-old started limping a couple of days ago.
When should we start worrying?***

Maybe now. You should take a child with a limp seriously. We do. Let's start with what we mean by a "limp."

A limp is a jerky, uneven gait that's usually caused by pain, muscle weakness, or, if chronic, some sort of deformity. Because it started only a couple of days ago, this isn't chronic, so we can narrow our focus on what might be causing it. The good news is that most of the time the cause is benign and the limp will quickly improve. A limp is usually brought on by some kind of minor trauma; it's the other causes that concern us.

> "Pay attention to your child. Without words, they will speak to you."
>
> **AUTHOR UNKNOWN**

Limps come in several different kinds, and they're based on where the problem lies. Watching your child carefully as she walks will give us important clues, and two types of limp are especially helpful in making a diagnosis. The first is straightforward—when a child quickly hops after planting her foot on the floor. That usually locates the affected *side* of the problem because the pain of pressure in that leg makes her want to get off of it. The pain could be anywhere—hip, knee, foot, ankle.

If the pain is coming from the hip, another type of limp can help localize the problem. This limp presents a downward *tilt* of one side of the pelvis, and the downward side is where the problem lies. We'll talk in a while about what can cause that, but watch your child walk and study his limp. Keep in mind that three- to four-year-olds normally walk in a peculiar fashion. They typically flex their hips, knees, and ankles, keeping a lower center of gravity and more balance. In addition, their feet normally splay out a little, and they walk faster, with shorter strides. That's not a limp. They didn't walk this way when they were two, and they won't when they're five.

Once we've established the presence of a limp, we ask a bunch of questions.

- *How long has this been going on?* A recent onset (several days) is typical of trauma or an acute infection. A longer duration (gradually increasing over weeks or months) is suspicious for overuse problems or certain types of hip pathology.

- *Has there been any recent trauma?* We're interested in minor falls, contusions, or sprains. Something called a "toddler's fracture" can occur with minimal or even unnoticed trauma, and if you have a child in that age range, we need to keep this in mind. If your child has older siblings (who might have been involved in some unsanctioned rough-housing), their historical accounts are not always going to be accurate.

- *Has there been any recent fever?* This is important because fever can be a red flag for the presence of two serious problems—an infected joint or an active bone infection.

- *What's the pain like?* We all need to be patient here because some children aren't able to articulate an answer to this question, and most children can't even accurately locate their pain. They just point to the entire extremity. (That goes for a lot of adults as well.) But the type of pain will tell us a lot. Constant, localized pain is seen with fractures, joint infections, and bone infections. Pain that's less severe and comes and goes is what we see with some degenerative hip problems (more about that later). Pain that worsens with activity might be coming from a stress fracture or overuse injury. Pain that occurs at night or awakens your child from sleep is another red flag. This might suggest the presence of a boney tumor, either benign or malignant. And if a young child refuses to walk and will only crawl on his knees, the problem is frequently in the feet. One last point about pain: "Referred pain" can confuse and mislead patients and physicians alike. Your child complains of knee pain, but the X-ray shows her knee is completely normal. The problem resides in her hip, but the pain is "referred" to the knee. That's commonly seen in adults as well. We're not sure why, but this happens a lot.

After we get a detailed history, we take a good look at your child, locate the site of his pain, and more than likely order some X-rays. Most experts recommend getting "plain" X-rays if your child has a definite limp, even in the presence of some kind of minor trauma. (Some studies have found that as many as 1 in 5 children will have a subtle fracture in this circumstance, which we don't want to miss.)

Blood work might be needed as well, but most often, that's not the case. However, if we find any of those red flags (fever, swollen joints, boney tenderness, or pain that occurs at night, among others), we might need to order some studies. Focused blood work will help us identify infection and inflammation. Generally, this won't be necessary if your child has no fever; there's been only a minor, isolated injury; or the limp has been present for less than 24 hours.

If we're still concerned after the initial X-rays, an ultrasound might be helpful, or even an MRI. Occasionally, if a specific joint is involved, it might need to be aspirated (joint fluid drawn through a needle), with the fluid studied for evidence of a joint-destroying infection. This is painful but necessary. And it should be done by an orthopedist.

A word about X-rays: While we want to limit your child's exposure to radiation, it's frequently necessary to get comparison views—X-rays of both hips, for example. Subtle findings might be missed with only one side examined. Or what appears to be a problem on the right side can also be present on the left side, hence a normal variation and not of significance.

We've noted some red flags here, so let's consider a few of the serious problems we could be facing.

An *infected joint* is an emergency. Undiagnosed and untreated, this infection can lead to a whole host of problems with lifelong consequences. Children with this problem will typically have a fever and appear quite sick. The knee and hip are the joints most often affected, with the hip most often involved in infants and young children.

A *bone infection* (osteomyelitis) is another emergency, and they usually occur in children younger than five. The diagnosis can be difficult because fever isn't always present and the symptoms can be nonspecific—dull pain, swelling, maybe some redness, and a history of minor trauma/contusion or a seemingly insignificant puncture wound. Your physician will need to maintain a high level of suspicion.

*Slipped capital epiphysis* is one of the most common hip problems in the middle-school years and in teenagers. It develops gradually, is associated with being overweight, and presents with dull, achy pain and a limp. There's no trauma involved and no fever. The problem lies in the growth plate of the hip, which "slips" off to one side. You can see this on an X-ray, but the longer it's out of place and the more it's slipped, the greater the potential for a lasting problem. This needs the attention of an orthopedist.

*Aseptic necrosis of the hip* is the last thing we want to consider in this chapter. You might know it as Legg-Calve-Perthes disease. Don't let the name fool you. This isn't some rare problem that's only of interest to medical students taking exams. We saw two cases of this just in the past month. Something happens to the blood flow to the hip, and the head of the hip eventually collapses. The peak incidence for this is between five and seven years of age, more boys than girls are affected (by a ratio of about 4:1), and it can occur on *both* sides in up to 1 in 5 children. Interestingly, African-American children are rarely affected. The cause is unknown, and any pain will be mild. A limp will develop, the one we described with the affected hip tilting downward. Early diagnosis is crucial, along with management by an experienced orthopedist. Again, we've seen two cases in the past month. It's out there.

So, yes, if your child starts to limp, pay attention. Here's what we recommend:

- A toddler with a limp should be checked.
- If your child's leg won't bear any weight at all, someone needs to see him.
- If there's been no trauma, no fever, no swelling, no redness, and no joint involvement, then watchful waiting is probably safe—but only for 24 hours.
- Everything else (know your red flags) needs attention.

*"Be alert. The most important things in life*
*are seldom the most obvious."*

Jonathan Lockwood Huie

# SIDS

✛ *My husband and I are expecting our first child
in two months, and it seems that someone's talking
about SIDS in every prenatal class we attend.
Is SIDS something we should be worried about?*

Worried about it? No. But you need to be aware of it. Sudden Infant Death Syndrome (SIDS), sometimes referred to as "sudden unexpected infant death," is one of the most traumatic and catastrophic things that can happen to young parents and their entire family.

The sudden loss of a previously healthy infant is devastating, and the more we know about what causes it and how to keep it from happening, the better off we'll be. We've learned a lot about SIDS over the past two or three decades, and with this knowledge has been a significant reduction in its incidence. Yet even one child dying from SIDS is too many. The American Academy of Pediatrics (AAP) has been at the forefront in addressing this issue, and in this chapter we will draw largely from their recommendations.

> "I cannot think of anyone stronger than a mother who has lost her child...and still breathes."
>
> **ROBYNA MAY**

First, we need to define the term "SIDS." SIDS is the sudden death of an infant younger than one year of age that remains unexplained after a thorough investigation of the case and a complete autopsy and examination of the death scene. This is important, because other possible causes of death—cardiac issues, infections, undiagnosed congenital problems—won't be uncovered without this complete investigation. We know of several families whose incapacitating sense of guilt was relieved when they learned the death of their child wasn't caused by anything they did or didn't do. Rather, the cause was a subtle congenital finding that would have been difficult to find and impossible to treat. So there's the need for a complete review and, as painful and difficult as it might be, a complete autopsy.

But how common is SIDS? SIDS is the leading cause of infant mortality between one month and one year of age in the United States. The risk in the US is a little less than 1 per 1,000 live births in white children, but two to three times that number in black and Native American children. And while we used to think it was much more common in boys, we now know the risk in males is only slightly more than it is in females.

We mentioned that the upper age limit seems to be one year. Current evidence indicates that the median age for SIDS deaths is about 11 weeks (*median* means that as many SIDS deaths occur with infants younger than 11 weeks as occur with older infants), and the peak incidence is between two and four months. Ninety percent of SIDS deaths occur before six months of age, and only 2 percent occur after nine months. That's good information, and it lets us know when we need to be most vigilant.

Now let's consider the risk factors since they're what we want to eliminate or at least try to manage. We'll start with those related to the mother.

- *Young maternal age.* This means the mother is under 20, and while we can't change it, it's a risk factor, and we need to be aware of it.

- *Maternal smoking.* This factor is especially concerning during pregnancy but also during the newborn period and beyond. (We know secondhand smoke confers significant risk as well.)

- *Late or no prenatal care.* Every expectant young woman should be actively and repeatedly encouraged to have regular prenatal visits. This is the best opportunity for education and for modifying dangerous behavior.

- *Alcohol and substance abuse.* These are two of those dangerous behaviors just mentioned, and we know them to be risk factors for SIDS.

Next, lets consider the infant and environmental factors we know to be risks:

- *Preterm birth and/or low birth weight.* These terms are defined as less than 37 weeks gestation and less than five and a half pounds at birth. The increased risk is somewhere between three and five times. Optimal prenatal care can help reduce the incidence of prematurity.

- *Prone sleeping position* (sleeping on your tummy). This is the big one! It's the strongest modifiable risk factor of SIDS because the odds ratio can approach a multiplier of 13. That means if you put your infant to sleep on her tummy, you've multiplied her chances of dying from SIDS by 13 times. We've known this for a while, and yet some parents apparently are not aware of its importance. Avoidance of side positioning is also important because the possibility of rolling from the side to the prone position is greater than that of rolling from the supine position to the prone position.

- *Sleeping on a soft surface with soft bedding accessories.* How important is this factor? When the prone position is combined with the use of soft bedding, the risk of SIDS rises by a factor of 21! So what is considered soft bedding? Examples include sheepskin bedding, a sofa or recliner, air mattresses, polystyrene beads, and natural fiber mattresses. A firm sleeping surface is best. And loose blankets, pillows, quilts, stuffed toys, and sheepskins should be avoided. This is especially true as the infant becomes older and can roll onto the soft objects, creating a risk of suffocation.

- *Bed sharing.* Infants sleeping in bed with their parents are at an increased risk of SIDS. This is greatest for those younger than three months of age or for infants of mothers who smoke. This is different from "room sharing," which the AAP encourages, especially if the mother is breastfeeding.

- *Overheating.* This risk increases with the amount of clothing or blankets placed on an infant, along with a higher room temperature. The mechanism for this risk is not well understood, but it has been established. Overheating— from whatever cause—should be monitored and avoided.

- *Swaddling.* This will come as a surprise to many, but swaddling appears to increase the risk of SIDS, especially for older infants and those not placed on their back to sleep. While swaddling might be safe in very young infants, as children grow older and attempt to roll over, they can move into an unsafe sleeping position. If you're determined to swaddle your child, talk to your pediatrician and get his guidance.

- *Having a sibling who died with SIDS.* Siblings of SIDS victims have an increased risk, but in most families, that risk remains less than 1 percent.

An important point to keep in mind is that 95 percent of SIDS victims have at least one of these risk factors. That's why we need to be familiar with all of them and put our knowledge to use.

What about protective measures? What can we do to help reduce the risk of SIDS in our young children? First, of course, we need to avoid all of the risk factors noted above. The most important is to *put your children on their back to sleep!* That can't be stressed enough. And we can do these other things to help lower the risk:

- *Room sharing.* We mentioned this earlier, and it's something to consider. It seems that having the infant sleep in close proximity to the mother supports breastfeeding (see below) and having the infant in the room with the parents reduces the risk of SIDS. This is *room* sharing and not *bed* sharing, and the benefit doesn't extend to sharing a room with other children.[1]

- *Breastfeeding.* Several studies have shown that breastfeeding for at least two months cuts the risk of SIDS in half.

- *Pacifier use.* The AAP suggests offering a pacifier during sleep as long as it doesn't interfere with establishing successful breastfeeding.

- *Using a fan in the room.* We're not sure how this works, but increased air movement around an infant reduces the risk of SIDS.

Here are a couple of other important points:

- *Immunizations are* not *associated with an increased risk of SIDS.* Up-to-date immunizations might even lower the risk.

- *Home monitors have no proven benefit.* Save your money. These things don't work.

So back to that original question...Should you worry about SIDS? No. But you need to keep this information in mind, eliminate the risk factors you can, and enjoy your new baby.

> *"That the birds of worry and care fly over your head,*
> *this you cannot change,*
> *but that they build nests in your hair,*
> *this you can prevent."*
>
> Chinese Proverb

# 23

# Palpitations

✚ *Our teenage boy says his heart feels like it's flipping over,*
*and he has palpitations. What's going on?*
*And what should we do?*

First, we're dealing with a symptom or feeling and not a specific diagnosis. The term "palpitation" describes a noticeable heartbeat that's perceived by the patient and causes concern. These palpitations can be fast, too strong, or irregular. We need to make a distinction between palpitations in an adult, which can frequently be the first sign of a serious heart condition, and those occurring in children, which usually arise from bodily reactions. Palpitations can be a response to fever, anxiety, strenuous exercise, and sometimes a significant and previously unnoticed anemia.

The good news is that most often the complaint of palpitations in a child or teenager is nothing serious. The exception is if your child has a history of heart disease, heart surgery, or unexplained blackout spells. That's a different story, and palpitations in those settings require an evaluation by a pediatric cardiologist. But you should already know about that and have a plan of action. Here we're going to consider what to do with the previously healthy youngster who complains of a funny feeling in her chest and describes what feels like palpitations.

So what might that complaint sound like? She might describe a feeling of "butterflies in my chest" or say that her heart is "beating so fast it feels like it's going to burst out of my chest." These episodes usually last seconds to a few minutes. Another description might be a pounding or rushing in her ears, especially when lying down. This can be from a hyperdynamic state—her cardiac output has increased significantly enough to be perceived. Or this can be a result of fever, exercise, certain drugs, anemia, too much caffeine, or emotional stress. This hyperdynamic state can last from minutes to hours.

And, finally, there's that sensation that a heart is "flipping over." You might have felt this yourself. Most of us have, and it's usually caused by an extra heartbeat. The heart pauses after the extra beat, and the chambers fill more than usual, causing the next beat to push more blood into the system. Some people—including children—can be very sensitive to this and describe the heart as flipping over or even stopping. These extra beats are common and are usually nothing to worry about. We'll talk about when to worry a little later. First, let's consider how your physician should approach this problem.

As always, a careful and complete history is important. Palpitations that stop and start abruptly—like a light switch being turned on and off—can suggest a potentially worrisome problem. These episodes usually last only seconds to a few minutes. The sensation of "my heart is flipping over" can be a result of the extra beats we considered earlier. One type of these extra beats—a premature ventricular contraction (PVC)—can be completely normal, though it can sometimes indicate cardiac irritability. And palpitations that result in a loss of consciousness are always a cause for concern. So with the history, doctors need to know what your child is feeling when this happens and what she was doing when it started. How did she look and how did she act?

Several vital sign changes can be important. A heartbeat that is too fast or too slow is one of those signs. A child's heartbeat should generally fall in these ranges:

- less than two years of age—90 to 160 BPM
- two to ten—70 to 140 BPM
- over ten, teenagers, and young adults—60 to 100 BPM

A good of rule of thumb is that if your child's heartbeat is too fast to count, it's probably over 180 BPM.

This is a good time to stress the importance of being able to accurately assess your own pulse as well as that of your child. You can check it over your wrist (over the radial artery), or better yet, over the carotid artery in your neck. Light pressure is all you need, and only one side at a time! It's okay to time the beats for 30 seconds and multiply by two, but no fewer. A full minute will give you a more accurate measurement, and you might pick up some of those extra beats. It's also a good idea to write this down, along with the time and date. Practice this when you're feeling fine so you're comfortable doing it under stress.

What's the next step? A careful and complete physical exam is in order, and then an electrocardiogram (ECG) should be done. Depending on the history, physical, and ECG, some focused blood work might also be called for. A CBC (complete blood count) will point us to a potential infection or anemia, and a blood sugar test might detect previously undiagnosed diabetes. Less frequently, thyroid studies confirm a diagnosis of an overactive thyroid gland.

If all of this testing checks out with no concerning findings, outpatient follow-up is indicated, maybe involving a 24-hour cardiac monitor. If there was any documented blackout—even in the face of a normal exam and ECG—or if your child has a history of congenital heart disease or cardiac surgery, insist on getting a pediatric cardiologist involved.

While we have to approach the complaint of palpitations with caution, it's important to keep in mind that the majority of children who experience them have a simple and benign condition. Make sure your child is evaluated thoroughly. And then relax.

And learn to take a pulse!

*"Take care of your body.*
*It's the only place you have to live."*

Jim Rohn

# 24

# Tics

**✚ My ten-year-old has started squeezing his eyes closed while scrunching his shoulders. My best friend says it's probably a tick, but my son hasn't been out in the woods or anything. What could it be?**

Ah, the English language—purported to be the most difficult to learn in all the world. Consider the confusion of someone trying to differentiate between a homophone and a homonym. You can list a bunch of homophones: to, too, two; so, sew; be, bee; principals, principles. They can be fun but confusing. Homonyms might be even worse. The spelling's the same, but how do you know which is intended—a noun or a verb—when you see or hear these words: bark, bolt, nails, pool, mine.

This is true in medicine as well. Vein or vain? Heal or heel? Die or dye? Muscle or mussel? Jugular or juggler? Gotta get these straight. But that's tough, and a homonym was what almost did one of us in. He'll go nameless, but he spent more than 25 years in the ER and should have known better.

On a Saturday night in the distant past, this doc found himself in a busy ER being swamped by a never-ending rush of patients. He decided to take the situation in hand and went out into the waiting area (always a mistake). There, with clipboard in hand, he began triaging a row of seated patients. He came to a young man who was sitting cross-legged and clutching a dish towel to his lower leg.

"What happened?" queried the doctor.

"Got hit by a bat," was the terse response.

The doctor passed a scribbled note to the unit secretary, and within minutes the young patient was taken around the corner to radiology for X-rays of his lower leg. A baseball bat can do a lot of damage.

Thirty minutes later, one of the radiology techs called the ER doc and asked, "Are you sure you want an X-ray of this man's leg?"

"Of course. He got hit by a bat."

A pause, and then, "Doctor, he got hit by a *flying* bat. The vampire kind. Skin's not broken or anything."

Another pause, and then, "Go ahead and cancel that. I'll find out who ordered it."

Again, that was a long time ago, and learning took place. The point was never forgotten, and it was a constant reminder that we have to pay attention to our words. The same is true here. This mother's best friend suggested the presence of a "tic," not a "tick," and she was probably right. We need to know about tics and try to understand them.

Tics are intermittent, repeated movements usually specific to the individual child. We can classify them as being "simple" (head jerking, blinking, facial grimacing, or shoulder shrugging) or "complex" (kicking, jumping, a bizarre gait, or strange body gyrations). The majority of tics fall into the simple category and are transient—meaning they last less than one year. They're common (as many as 1 in 10 normal children might be affected), and if truth be told, many of us have experienced this problem ourselves. That might be a blessing, because then we'll have insight into what's going on with our children and be able to share our own experiences with them.

### ✚ Aren't tics voluntary? I mean, doesn't my child cause them to happen? Can't children control them?

Not exactly. Most experts describe simple tics as being semivoluntary or "unvoluntary," but not voluntary. Is that clear enough? Hmm. The reason for this less-than-clear explanation is that your child might be able to suppress an urge to perform his tic, but only for a brief time.

The tic will occur, followed by a sense of relief. Then the clock resets. We call it simple, but it's not. Here are some things we know about simple tics:

- They frequently start before the age of three.
- To officially be termed a tic, the performance needs to be present for at least three months.
- As mentioned above, tics can be suppressed but only temporarily (this is important regarding treatment).
- Tics decrease when a child is focused on something and increase with stress, anxiety, and fatigue (another important treatment point).
- Tics don't occur during sleep.
- The presence of other conditions alongside tics is common, the most frequent being obsessive compulsive disorder (OCD), ADHD, and anxiety.
- Tics are preceded by an identifiable urge or sensation (another help with treatment).
- A "tic storm" can happen after a day at school or other outing when a child has worked hard to suppress a tic. Once back home or in another nonthreatening environment, an explosive presence of his tic is called a "storm." It will pass.

### ✛ How can I help my child?

Start with understanding the problem and then exercising patience. That's key—*patience*. We'll focus on the approach to what we call simple tics because those are actually the more complex tics (Tourette's Syndrome is one), and they need to be addressed by trained and experienced counselors. Here's what we recommend:

- Look at the Yale Global Tic Severity Scale (YGTSS) or the Premonitory Urge for Tics Scale (PUTS). They're not nearly as intimidating as they sound, and they'll provide both information and a way to assess the significance and severity of your child's tic. Understanding comes first.

- Make it your goal not to confront or threaten/intimidate your child when you notice the tic. She can't help it.

- Ensure that your child is getting adequate and good-quality sleep.

- Try to identify causes of stress and deal with them.

- Educate other family members about this condition and about your plans for intervention.

- Talk with your child openly, but don't draw excessive attention to the tic. Be positive: "We're going to work through this."

- If your child is old enough, try to identify his trigger feelings. What does he feel/sense before the onset of the tic? Can he describe it?

With these points in mind, we can develop a strategy to help. The strategy is initially based on "behavior therapy." If you've identified the trigger or warning sign, have a plan of action for your child, like deep breathing or focused attention on some other activity (such as clenching and unclenching a fist with the hand in her pocket). This is a form of "habit reversal therapy" (HRT), which involves three components: awareness training, competing response training, and social support. You might be able to do this at home, but a more formal intervention might be available with trained therapists. Give it a try. And, again, be patient.

"Have patience...I am currently under construction."

**YOUR CHILD**

If behavior therapy isn't successful, you have another option: medication. But although some medications have proven to be of benefit, they have some bothersome side effects. Medication is a last resort and is seldom needed with simple tics. Remember, these usually go away within a year, most within a few weeks or months. They can recur, though, and occasionally they do so with a completely different presentation. Again, most will go away after a few months. If your physician immediately reaches for a prescription pad, call a time-out. And remember, it's a "tic" not a "tick."

Sew weather or not ewe will ever sea won of these, keep this inn mined: Bee aware of watt tics look like, no wen two get help, and remember you herd and red about them hear.

*"Have patience.*
*All things are difficult before they become easy."*

Saadi

# 25

# Foreign Bodies in Noses

✚ *Junior is three years old, and he put a bead in his nose.*
*I can see it, but I can't get it out. Should I take him to the ER?*

Not just yet. Let's try something first.

"You're out of your mind. You know that, right?"

Lori Davidson was leaning close and whispering in my ear. She was the nurse helping me with the young child in our ENT room. The boy sat on his mother's lap, staring at the two of us with wide, frightened eyes. I ignored Lori's comments and repeated my instructions to his mother.

> "Most children threaten at times to run away from home. This is the only thing that keeps some parents going."
>
> **PHYLLIS DILLER**

The ER chart had read, "Four-year-old with foreign body in nose." This was a common problem, and the foreign body could be something simple or something that could leave us all frustrated and the boy on the way to the OR for removal while under sedation.

Sometimes it turns out to be nothing. An anxious parent thought he saw his child playing with a small object before putting her hand to her face or nose, and then the object disappeared. It had to go somewhere, and if she hadn't swallowed it, kids were pretty good at hiding things in their noses. We're not sure why that happens, but it does—a lot. When a careful exam doesn't reveal any nasal foreign body, we're all relieved.

Not so with four-year-old Stevie. I could see what appeared to be a round, blue bead—a little bigger than a BB—lodged in his left nostril. His mother confirmed the size and shape of the missing object and confessed that she might have pushed it further into his nose when she tried to remove it with some tweezers.

"That's okay," I had reassured her. "No harm done, and it's always worth a try."

The fact that the bead was round was good news. While it wouldn't present an edge or unusual shape to grasp with ENT forceps, the presence of an edge frequently prevents an easy extraction. What might have gone into a nostril with ease could hang up with a reverse movement. Stevie had done us a favor by choosing a round foreign body.

"Okay, Mama, do you understand what to do?" I asked her, moving back a little on the rolling stool.

"I...think so." She hesitated for only a moment, and then she swung Stevie around so that he remained on her lap but now faced her head-on. "Like this?" She placed a finger on the right side of Stevie's nose and closed that nostril.

"Great," I told her. "Now take a breath and blow in his mouth."

Out of the corner of my eye, I could see Lori shaking her head.

Stevie's mother took a breath, leaned close to her boy, and blew into his mouth.

Nasal secretions (you might call it something else) flew out of his left nostril and into his mother's face. Along with it came the bead, flying through the air before landing on the floor and rolling out of sight.

Stevie was unfazed, and I handed his mother some Kleenex. I had warned her about what to expect, but she was willing to try anything to help her child. Only a mother's love.

A few weeks later, I was walking down the hallway and passed the door into ENT. Lori was in the room standing behind one of our younger ER docs. "That's right," she was instructing him. "Just have the mother pinch the other side of his nose and then blow into his mouth. It'll work, I promise."

Well, not always, though I'm now 10 for 10 with this method. It's not very exotic, but it's worth a try before going to the ER or your doctor's office. The bottom line is that if your child puts something in her nose, it needs to come out. It's always helpful to know what we're dealing with—size and shape, sometimes even color. And always check the other nostril.

Oh, and take a peek in those ears. For whatever reason, kids can be packrats.

*"If evolution really works,*
*how come mothers only have two hands?"*

Milton Berle

# 26

# Swimmer's Ear

### ✚ *What's the best thing for swimmer's ear?*

The best thing for swimmer's ear is not to get it. Really, we're serious. This is one of those conditions that's preventable if we just pay attention and use a little common sense.

Let's start by considering the causes of the problem—technically known as *otitis externa*. This is an inflammation or infection of the ear canal, the one-inch tube that leads to the eardrum. Behind the eardrum is the middle ear, the site of *otitis media*—the infection that plagues most of our young children at some point and even those of us who pretend to be adults.

*Otitis externa* occurs in all age groups but is most common during childhood (ages 5 to 15), and it's more likely to be experienced during the summer months. For some reason, the pain frequently presents in the middle of the night, waking both the child and parents. Or it can start earlier and prevent everyone from going to sleep. While the condition can be caused by inflammation or irritation (scratching, excessive cleaning, contact dermatitis), it's most frequently caused by a bacterial infection. The most frequent cause of that infection is water with bacteria from a pond, a lake, a swimming pool, an ocean, or even your shower that entered your ear and then stayed there.

Once in the ear, water, in combination with body heat and the darkness of the ear canal, creates a perfect environment for bacteria to grow. With any break in the natural defenses of the skin in the canal, these bacteria can penetrate that lining and cause an infection, resulting in mild, moderate, or serious symptoms. There's not much room in the canal for the soft tissue to expand, and any swelling quickly becomes painful. A mild infection involves only minimal inflammation and swelling and slight discomfort, but this can progress to a full-blown, serious infection, manifested by significant pain, swelling to the point of closing the ear canal, swollen lymph nodes around the ear, fever, and considerable pain. If you've ever had such an infection, you know what we're talking about, and it's no fun.

Treatment is straightforward and includes three important things:

1. *Cleaning the ear canal.* This is the first step, and it needs to be done carefully and not at home. If your child has a history of tubes or a perforated eardrum, the rules change, and you'll need to see your pediatrician or ENT specialist. The ear canal should be directly visualized, and any excess cerumen (earwax) or debris should be carefully removed. The canal can also be irrigated with a 1:1 solution of water and hydrogen peroxide, warmed to body temperature.

2. *Appropriate topical medications—ear drops.* Ear drops should contain an antibiotic that is active against the most common bacteria seen with these infections and a steroid component for swelling and inflammation. Sometimes your physician will need to place a wick in the canal. This is sponge-like material, and once it's inserted and soaked with the antibiotic drops, it will expand and allow the medication to reach the sides of the canal. This wick might need to be changed every couple of days, but once the swelling subsides, it will usually drop out on its own. Now about those ear drops. There's a right way to administer them and probably a bunch of wrong ways. The best technique is to have your child lie on his side for four or five minutes after the drops are instilled. Another option is to place a cotton ball in the ear canal for 20 minutes after the drops. We prefer keeping children down for a couple of minutes because a significant amount of the drops soaks into the cotton and does no good. And make sure you use

the right number of drops. Follow the directions, because underdosing is the leading cause of treatment failure.

3. *Pain control.* Pain is usually controlled with acetaminophen or ibuprofen along with carefully applied dry heat (a closely monitored heating pad).

You should see a big improvement in 36 to 48 hours. If not, you might want to give your doctor a call and have your child rechecked. But by two days, most of us are better.

Many parents ask about an oral antibiotic because this is an ear infection. In this case, oral antibiotics don't help. The exception is a severe infection with fever, facial swelling, and significant pain. Those cases are rare and are usually treated in a hospital setting.

### ✚ My granny used to put sweet oil in my ear when I was a child and had an earache. It always seemed to help. What have you got to say about that?

Well, we don't want to argue with Granny, but if the oil helped, you probably didn't have an infection. Warmed sweet oil (usually this means olive oil) can provide temporary relief for ear pain, but it won't clear an infection, and it usually makes it difficult for a doctor to get a good look at the canal and eardrum. If your child is having bad enough pain for you to consider doing this with oil, that's a good indication that you should have her examined.

Now, about the prevention of this problem. Because the most common cause of swimmer's ear is water in the ear canal, we need to keep that water from getting in there in the first place or remove it should it find its way there. We've all gotten water in our ears at some point—swimming, showering—and we know how difficult it can be to get out. Tilting your head to one side and jumping up and down won't do it. Nor will pounding on the side of your head. The water just trickles back. It has to come out, and here's a quick and simple technique.

Take a half-capful of rubbing alcohol, have your child lie on her side, pour the alcohol in the ear, and count to five. Then flip her over and repeat. This works every time, and while some encouragement might be needed, it isn't painful. (Remember, this shouldn't be done if your child has tubes or a known perforation.)

Do this anytime your children have been swimming. Whether it's in your pool, in the ocean, or in someone's lake doesn't matter. Bugs are everywhere. Make this a habit, and you'll avoid many, if not all, of those late-night summertime cries of, "Mommy, my ear hurts."

> *"An ounce of prevention* [really!] *is worth a pound of cure."*
>
> Benjamin Franklin

27

# Cat and Dog Bites

✢ *Which is worse, a dog or a cat bite?*
*And when should we worry about it?*

If you had thrown in *human bite,* that would have been the clear "worse" winner. In James 3:6, the apostle tells us that the tongue is "a world of evil" that adversely affects the rest of our bodies. While he was operating on a more spiritual level, it remains true that the human tongue and mouth are indeed "evil" when it comes to the presence of multiple bacteria that can cause a host of problems. That's also true of dogs and cats; a human bite can just be far worse. But let's get back to the question above and start with cat bites.

## Cat Bites

A cat's bite can cause serious problems, usually much worse than a bite from a dog. Not only do cats harbor different and more hostile bacteria than dogs do, but their bites can seem minor at first—maybe only several innocuous puncture wounds. Don't be fooled. Bacteria driven deep into our soft tissues can quickly take hold and cause a significant infection. This is especially true for wounds to the hands and legs—favorite targets for these carnivores. And injuries to the face can cause lifelong cosmetic challenges.

✢ *Is this the same as "cat scratch fever"?*

Some people do call this infection cat scratch fever, but that's the title of a song by Ted Nugent, and this infection is usually referred to as cat scratch disease. Cat scratch disease is a common problem following a cat scratch or bite. Most affected are children and young adults, and the problem is seen most frequently on the hands and arms. This infection is caused when a specific type of bacteria enters the skin, forms a localized lesion, and spreads to a nearby lymph node, causing it to swell. That's the trademark of this problem, with the swelling noted about two weeks after the bite or scratch and enlarging to as much as two inches in diameter. This infection needs to be treated with antibiotics, which shorten its course from four months to about three weeks and reduce the risk of more serious complications, such as eye problems, nervous system injuries, and liver and spleen infections. Cat scratch disease is nothing to mess around with.

## Dog Bites

Now let's consider dog bites, whether the dog is your own pet, a neighbor's dog, or a stray wandering down the street. These wounds need attention. Larger dogs have strong jaws and large teeth, causing substantial skin and soft tissue damage, and the threat of infection is ever present. Hands and fingers are especially problematic—with the potential for long-term scarring and contracture—and, of course, facial injuries in a child scare all of us. The face of a young child is at a large dog's mouth level, and as parents we need to always be watchful. But should a bite occur, it has lifelong implications, and your child deserves the best of care. Insist on it.

The treatment of these wounds needs to be aggressive, including a complete examination of the areas around the bite, a thorough cleansing with something that kills bugs, consideration of the use of a prophylactic antibiotic, and the judicious implementation of wound closure (sutures). Conventional wisdom, wherever it came from, is that none of these wounds should be closed because doing so will most likely lead to a serious infection. But just washing out the bite, covering it, and letting it heal on its own is not a proven treatment. That's the easy way out for the health care provider and the bad way out for the patient.

Unless over the hands and fingers, or in the presence of diabetes or large and severely damaged tissue, these bites can be carefully sutured and observed closely. This almost always results in much quicker healing times and less scarring, important considerations for young patients, especially those with facial injuries. If your health care provider doesn't offer sutures, ask him why. And maybe ask him what he would do for his child.

Regarding the use of oral antibiotics for these injuries, we routinely recommend them for cat bites (always for cat scratch disease) and usually for dog bites, though this can be a case-by-case consideration, depending on the size and depth of the wound.

### ✚ When do we worry about rabies?

The possibility of rabies is another important consideration, especially when dealing with a stray dog or cat. In most states, health care providers are required to report these bites to an animal control agency, and then these individuals investigate the circumstances and recommend appropriate follow-up, including the need for rabies vaccination. Note that this is required, and while sometimes aggravating in the heat of the moment, it's a helpful service from men and women who are simply doing their job.

The bottom line is that every dog or cat bite or scratch should be taken seriously. Don't wait around to see what happens.

*"Caution is the parent of safety."*

Author Unknown

# 28

# Slapped Cheek Disease

✚ *My seven-year-old came home from school
with beet-red cheeks and a note from his teacher
that said it looks like fifth disease. What's that?
And should I worry about the sixth and seventh?*

Wow! One of our grandchildren just had this problem. It was a week before Christmas, and this grandchild was sent home from school with a fever, a cough, and bright-red cheeks. Turns out the community was in the early stages of a citywide outbreak of *erythema infectiosum*—more commonly known as "slapped cheek disease" or fifth disease. We'll talk about this "fifth" business in a moment, but first we need to understand this particular infection.

Slapped cheek disease is another of those problems whose name does a good job of describing the physical findings. This is caused by a parvovirus (if you're taking names), and it most often occurs in outbreaks among school-aged children, though it can occur in adults as well. It's highly contagious and starts with nonspecific symptoms, including a low-grade fever, congestion, headache, and even nausea and diarrhea. Two to five days later, the classic bright-red rash appears on the cheeks. There may even be some pallor around the mouth, which can accentuate the facial rash.

The incubation period—from the time of exposure to the onset of the rash—is usually one to two weeks but can be as long as three weeks. The rash is what helps us with the diagnosis. In addition to the cheeks, this lacey-appearing rash can be seen on a child's upper arms and even on her trunk. By the time it appears, the child is probably feeling better and is no longer contagious. That's important to remember, because the rash can be impressive, even alarming. But at this stage, the child is no longer spreading the virus. That damage has already been done.

The good news is that this infection is almost always mild and doesn't lead to any significant complications. The treatment is supportive, with lots of fluids, rest, and ibuprofen or acetaminophen for fever or discomfort. The rash is going to last for a while—days to a week or so—but it will go away.

### ✚ Isn't there something I can put on his cheeks to make the rash go away quicker? Cortisone or something?

Nope. The rash is thought to be "immunologically mediated" (meaning it's coming from the inside), and no topical treatments will help. However, we need to be aware of a typical feature of these "slapped cheeks," and that's the rash's tendency to get worse with exposure to sunlight, a rising temperature, exercise, and even emotional stress. Not to panic, though. It's still going to go away.

"No fight is harder than the struggle against the thing you want most to believe."

**MARTHA ALBRAND**

Now, why the name "fifth disease"? We can tell you nothing exciting here. This common viral exanthem (an infection with a rash) was the *fifth* such disease to be identified. The first four? Here they are:

1. rubeola—red measles

2. scarlet fever (also scarlatina)—caused by a strep infection and still seen today

3. rubella—German measles

4. "scalded skin" disease—caused by a staph infection. Some people insert chicken pox in this position because it also comes with a rash and is seen much more frequently than scalded skin.

5. fifth disease (slapped cheek)

And yes, there's a sixth disease—*roseola infantum*. Fortunately, we've stopped at six. No seventh or eighth disease has been identified. Not yet, anyway.

> *"There are only two things a child will share willingly:*
> *communicable diseases and its mother's age."*
>
> Benjamin Spock

# 29

# Weight Gain

**✛ *My teenage daughter just can't seem to lose weight.
It's probably a glandular problem, right?***

Glandular? Probably not. We often hear this idea, along with, "It must be genetic," as reasons for that teenage daughter being overweight. For the great majority of us—both children and adults—maintaining a healthy weight is a simple equation: what calories we take in versus what calories we burn. If we consume more calories than we burn, we gain weight, simple as that. However, we need to consider a couple of things with that overweight teenager, especially considering that she's a girl.

Polycystic ovary syndrome (PCOS) is a relatively common problem affecting as many as 1 in 40 women. That would be about seven million females in this country. Women who have this syndrome include such luminaries as Emma Thompson, Victoria Beckham, and Jillian Michaels. We're not sure what causes this syndrome, but we know what it looks like.

Symptoms usually begin in adolescence and present as increased facial and body hair, moderate to severe acne, abnormal menstrual cycles, and obesity. It can also be associated with mood changes (frequent anxiety and depression), a diminished quality of life, and even with eating disorders, including binge eating.

The name *polycystic* comes from the ultrasound findings of an increased number of cysts (more than 12 on one or both ovaries), although the presence of these cysts is not required to make the diagnosis.

As many as 50 percent of these young women struggle with obesity.

When present, it's hard to manage and almost always "central" (the apple-shaped body image we've all heard and read about). A very real risk is that this central obesity can lead to heart disease, diabetes, and high blood pressure. That makes it important to consider this possibility, establish an accurate diagnosis, and if your daughter has this syndrome, start treatment.

The treatment for PCOS is effective and includes a commonly used and inexpensive medication, metformin. You might be familiar with it because it's a mainstay in the treatment of diabetes. This makes sense when we consider that young women with PCOS share some of the same problems as those with diabetes, including struggles handling glucose and having issues with insulin. Just as we're not sure what causes this problem, we're not exactly sure how metformin helps, but it does. And as a bonus, the use of metformin can result in weight loss and maintenance. So PCOS is treatable, but it has to be considered and then diagnosed.

The other condition to be considered with that overweight teenager *is* glandular—an underactive thyroid gland. While usually a disease of older individuals, it can be present in teenagers and rarely in younger children. If you're keeping score, as many as 5 percent of Americans have some degree of an underactive thyroid—hypothyroidism. You've heard of some of these people, including Linda Ronstadt, Oprah Winfrey, Sofia Vergara, Rod Stewart, Kelly Clarkson, and, historically, John Adams. In addition to obesity, it manifests itself with fatigue, cold intolerance, poor concentration and memory, thinning hair, and dry skin. Once diagnosed with simple blood work, the treatment is straightforward and effective. When corrected, those affected have more energy, feel a whole lot better, and usually lose weight.

So glandular? It's possible, but not very likely. The first thing to do is analyze that simple equation, and if your child needs to lose weight, make sure she's burning more calories than she's taking in.

*"Weight loss is not a physical challenge—it's a mental one."*

Author Unknown

# 30

# Hand, Foot, and Mouth Disease

### ✚ What do we need to know about hand, foot, and mouth disease?

Isn't it great when we have a disease whose name perfectly describes it? It makes communication a lot simpler than trying to remember some syndrome named after an obscure Lithuanian pathologist.

Most of us have seen, experienced, or at least heard of hand, foot, and mouth disease, so let's consider the most important points we should all know. HFMD was described only a few decades ago (1957), though the virus that causes it has been around for much longer. This is one of the Coxsackieviruses, a group that's capable of causing a wide range of infections in humans. This particular organism, an enterovirus, causes an infection after being orally ingested from either the GI tract or through upper respiratory secretions—the coughs and sneezes of an infected individual.

### ✚ A cough is one thing, but the GI tract?

That's right, the virus is ingested after we come into contact with infected fecal material. We know—that's pretty gross. But that's how it happens. Changing your child's dirty diaper is an opportunity just waiting to happen. What makes this important is that this virus is stable outside of the body. It can remain active and infectious for significant periods of time on a changing table, on bedclothes, or just about anywhere. Hence the need to clean and disinfect potentially contaminated areas.

Once ingested, the virus replicates in the GI tract and then spreads throughout the body. With HFMD, the incubation time from exposure to the appearance of the skin and mouth lesions is usually three to five days but can be up to one week. What makes this infection so difficult to contain is that a significant percentage of children can become infected but never have the rash. They can shed the virus through their GI tract for two or three months and through their respiratory tract for four weeks. This shedding can result in transmission to other children, who then can manifest the full-blown disease.

We expect to see this infection in late summer and early fall, and in children, particularly those younger than five to seven years of age. However, it can occur throughout the year and in any age group, even in adults. Interestingly, the skin lesions in teenagers and adults can be painful, unlike those in younger children.

What does HFMD look like? Let's start with the hands and feet. Typically, you'll see multiple raised, red, or blister-like lesions on the soles of feet, the backs of toes, the palms of hands, and the backs of fingers. These lesions are usually small—up to a quarter of an inch—but they can be larger. And while the hands and feet are most often involved, the rash can appear on the legs, the buttocks (frequently infants and young children), and even the face. These lesions don't itch, and as noted above, they usually aren't painful. Most are gone in three to four days.

The oral lesions look much the same and are generally found on the tongue, on the front and just outside the mouth, and inside the cheeks. A thin, red halo can surround the blisters, and they're about the same size as the skin lesions. With some types of this virus, these blisters can be painful and make eating and drinking difficult, especially for small children.

Here's the tricky part. While about 75 percent of patients have both the skin and mouth lesions, the other 25 percent have only one or the other. The diagnosis is made by the appearance of the rash and what's out there in the community. When HFMD is going through day-care facilities, schools, or any place where people gather, there will be a lot of infections.

In addition to the mouth and skin lesions and a sore throat, we expect to see only a low-grade temperature (less than 101) and not much else. This is almost always a benign and short-term problem. But we worry when a child develops a fever that persists for more than three days, starts vomiting, or won't eat or drink because of the painful mouth lesions (posing a significant risk of dehydration), or becomes lethargic. Those things need to be evaluated.

### ✚ What about treatment? Can't you do something?

The best care is supportive—plenty of fluids, ibuprofen or acetaminophen for pain and fever, and rest. Antibiotics won't do any good, and no antiviral medication is effective. The good news is that in the vast majority of those infected, HFMD is a nonthreatening process and resolves in a few days. But it is highly contagious, and that's something to keep in mind. While we're not completely sure, it appears that children are infectious for less than a week after the rash disappears. So wash your hands, keep your fingers out of your mouth, and disinfect that changing table!

*"Kids are like buckets of disease that live in your house."*

Louis C. K.

# 31

# Ticks

✚ *I found a tick on my four-year-old tonight*
*and panicked! It was crawling around on his back*
*and wasn't attached. What should I do?*

Why do you suppose these tiny arachnids inspire such fear and trembling? I don't have the answer, but I know they *do*. We see dozens of people in the ER each summer with a tick attached to their skin. And we see anxious parents who bring their child in with one embedded in their scalp—or maybe it's just crawling around. Sometimes they can't point out the creepy offender but want us to check the child just the same. And it's not just in the summertime. As I write this, it's December in South Carolina, and I found a tick crawling on my leg yesterday.

What do we do if we find one of these critters attached to our child's skin? There's one safe and effective method of removal and several bad ones.

Johnny Green sat on the ER stretcher, his legs dangling over the edge and swinging back and forth. His mother stood beside her four-year-old son with arms folded across her chest and head shaking.

"Mrs. Green, I'm Dr. Lesslie. What can we do for Johnny this afternoon?"

The complaint on his chart read "problem with scalp," which wasn't very helpful.

"Hmm," she responded, looking down at Johnny and shaking her head with impatient determination. "I should never have listened to my brother Jake," she huffed.

"*Uncle* Jake," Johnny said, correcting her.

"Well, your uncle Jake got you into this fix, and just where is he?"

"Hold on a second," I interjected. "What's the problem with Johnny's scalp?"

"It's more like the back of his head, and it started with a tick."

She unfolded her arms and stepped closer to the boy. He jumped as she fingered the back of his head.

"He had a tick bite?" I moved to one side of Johnny, trying to get a look at his scalp.

"That's right," she answered, not looking up from her examination. "Johnny is always outside in the woods, and he came in this morning scratching the back of his head. That's when I noticed the tick."

"Ow!" Johnny hollered, pulling back from his mother and blocking any chance I had of seeing whatever had necessitated this visit.

"That critter was stuck tight, and I tried to pull it off with my fingers. Well, that didn't work, so I tried using some of my daughter's eyebrow tweezers. No luck there either. That's when I remembered something I read about using kerosene. Didn't have any of that stuff, but I got some gasoline out of a can in the garage and dabbed some on. I waited a couple of minutes, but nothing happened. That's when Jake—*Uncle* Jake— walked in. I told him what was going on, and he reached in his pocket and pulled out a pack of matches. 'Here, try this match,' he said. 'Light it, blow it out, and while it's still good and hot, touch it to the back side of the tick. That'll get him movin'.'"

I knew what was coming next. Gently, I took the boy's head in my hands and examined his scalp.

"That's when Johnny's hair caught on fire," Mrs. Green said matter-of-factly. "Never seen that boy move faster in my life. He took off down the hall, hair on fire, and hollerin' loud enough to wake the dead."

No wonder. On the back of his head was a silver-dollar-sized area of singed hair and mildly blistered scalp. But no tick.

"Mrs. Green, let me tell you the best way to remove a tick the next time this happens."

In case you're still wondering, the best and safest way to remove a tick is to simply use some small, toothless tweezers. Gently grasp the body of the tick, pull slowly and gently, and you'll be successful. Don't squeeze the tweezers, because some people believe this might cause bacteria-laden saliva to be forced from the tick's mouth into the skin. Check closely to be sure the mouth parts (two small pinchers) are still attached to the tick, and you're done. If you're not sure they are, use some soap and water and a face cloth to do some scrubbing. Then take a close look again. If any doubt remains, it might be good to have your doctor take a look as well. This isn't a 9-1-1 call—24 to 48 hours is a safe window—but be aware of a couple of potential complications.

A simple skin infection can occur at the site of the bite. Telltale signs are swelling, redness, and maybe some drainage. More troubling is the potential for two serious infections—Rocky Mountain spotted fever (RMSF) and Lyme disease. RMSF is somewhat of a misnomer because this infection occurs throughout the country, not just west of the Rockies. We see it here in the Carolinas as well. And while Lyme disease was named after a town in Connecticut where it was first noted, deer have carried the offending organism far beyond the confines of the Northeast.

That brings up the issue of what to do if you child has a tick bite. Should she be given antibiotics or get some blood work done? And what about sending the tick (if you have it) to the state health department for testing? The last part is easy to answer. Most states (maybe all) are no longer testing ticks for RMSF or Lyme disease. The test is costly, takes too much time, and isn't all that accurate. The question of getting blood work is almost as easy. Immediate testing won't do any good. It's too soon for anything to turn up in your child's system, so this would be a waste of money and tears. The real question has to do with using a prophylactic antibiotic. In many parts of our country where these diseases are relatively common, it makes sense to give one or two doses of an appropriate medication that would prevent these illnesses. Good evidence exists that taking doxycycline (over the age of eight years) is safe and effective, as is amoxicillin for those children eight and younger. For those children who might be allergic to these drugs, other choices are available. The other option is watchful waiting, something most parents (me included) are not very good at.

If you find a tick on your child, reach for your tweezers and don't call Uncle Jake. No gasoline, no fire, and no scorched scalp.

*"Seek advice but use your own common sense."*

Yiddish Proverb

## 32

# Growing Pains

*✛ Our six-year-old wakes us up almost every night
with leg pains. Her grandmother says it's growing pains,
and I say there's no such thing.
Can you settle this for us? And tell us what to do?*

Well, her grandmother might be right. There *is* such a thing as growing pains, and it's pretty common. It's a diagnosis of *exclusion*, meaning there are no specific physical findings or diagnostic tests so you have to *exclude* other, more serious causes for those pains. Fortunately, the process of exclusion can be straightforward.

First, we need to define this problem as best we can, understanding there is no established consensus. What most experts (pediatricians, pediatric orthopedists, and pediatric rheumatologists) agree on are the following points:

- Growing pains wake children from sleep at night or from naps.
- They're likely present with no findings of any musculoskeletal problems and a physical exam that shows the child's condition is normal.
- They occur most commonly in preschool and school-aged children (ages 2 to 12).
- Up to 20 percent of children can be affected, and these growing pains are more common in girls than in boys.

- Growing pains are benign and usually resolve within a year or two of onset.

- Pain occurs primarily in the legs and is bilateral (in both legs).

- The pain is described as being deep and localized to the thigh or calf.

- The pain can be severe enough to cause the child to cry.

- Symptom-free periods are common, and they can last for days, weeks, or even months.

- Pain is usually relieved by massage, heat, or ibuprofen or acetaminophen.

- Up to one-third of children with growing pains will also have recurrent headaches and/or abdominal pain.

- There is frequently a family history of growing pains.

With these factors in mind, making a diagnosis of growing pains is almost always a clinical diagnosis, meaning it's based on a good history and a physical exam. Here's what we should see:

- Pain usually occurs late in the day or awakens the child from sleep.

- The pain isn't related to any joint.

- The pain is frequently worsened by increased physical activity during the day.

- Most experts expect the pain to occur at least once a month for at least three months.

- Again, the physical exam shows the child's physical condition is completely normal.

That's the key point here—the physical exam *must* be normal. Any of the following findings prompt further studies:

- unexplained fever, weight loss, or lack of energy/activity

- decreased range of motion of any joint, joint swelling, or tenderness directly over a bone
- abnormal and unusual skin changes
- a limp or signs of gait instability
- swollen lymph nodes
- pain during the day
- unilateral limb pain (on only one side)
- arm pain only with no leg pain

If any of these symptoms are present, the diagnosis of "growing pains" isn't appropriate. The list of other, more serious possibilities is long, and beyond the scope of what we're considering here. Once again, the physical exam should be completely normal if growing pains is what's going on, and that should be reassuring. Interestingly, about 50 percent of those experts we mentioned earlier would consider diagnostic studies in the child with probable growing pains even in the face of a normal exam. These will typically include plain X-rays of the involved extremity, a blood study that looks for evidence of inflammation, and a complete blood count, checking for any evidence of a bone marrow problem. All of these will be normal in a child with growing pains.

So once we're comfortable with this diagnosis, what are we to do? How do we help our six-year-old in the middle of the night? As previously mentioned, heat and gentle massage should help. And a measure of patience. Adults don't want to be awakened at three in the morning, but neither does a child. Patience and reassurance go a long way.

Regarding the use of medications, again, appropriate doses of ibuprofen or acetaminophen will usually control this pain. If your child has two or three episodes a week, consider giving the medicine before bed. If the episodes are more frequent, a longer-acting analgesic (naproxen) given in the evening may help prevent or at least lessen the intensity of the pain. None of these medications is to be used long term, and about a week is all we recommend. If the pain is worsening or is uncontrollable, it's probably time for another evaluation.

Along with patience and reassurance, another key to effective management of growing pains is to encourage your child's normal activities. Don't let these pains dominate you or your child's home life and emotions.

Yes, growing pains are real, but they can be managed, and they'll go away.

*"Pay heed to the tales of old wives.*
*It may be that they alone keep in memory*
*what it was once needful for the wise to know."*

J.R.R. Tolkien

## 33

# Ingrown Toenails

**✛ *My teenage boy keeps getting ingrown toenails.
What's the best thing to do, and can they be prevented?***

Yes, ingrown toenails can be prevented. But your son probably won't complain about one until his toe is markedly swollen and tender, and then he has to see your doctor. By then, the time for simple, conservative treatment has passed, and your doctor will need to do something more aggressive and probably painful. Get in the habit of checking your child's feet every couple of weeks or so, and you'll catch this before it gets too far along.

Ingrown toenails are way too common, and they usually involve the big toes. They start when a small, sharp piece of the nail burrows into the skin and causes inflammation, swelling, and pain. With enough time, they'll become infected and might start to drain. Frequent causes of this process are wearing too-tight shoes, improper nail trimming, and occasionally some mild trauma, such as a "stubbed toe." But by far the most common cause is improper trimming. Toenails should *never* be trimmed with fingernail clippers. *Never.* Fingernail clippers are curved and invite the edges of the toenail to dig into the skin border and start this process. Toenails should be trimmed with something straight and not trimmed too closely. The end of the nail should always be free of any skin or you're just inviting trouble. Invest in some toenail clippers, and make sure they're straight.

Now that you're going to check your child's toes every couple of weeks, what are you going to be looking for? Again, look for some redness and swelling along the edge of the nail and tenderness. Catch this early, and you can turn it around. Start with some warm, soapy water and soak the foot for 10 to 20 minutes three or four times a day. Sounds like a lot, and it is. But this will help. When the skin around the nail is soft from the soaking, gently push the edges back from the nail, a little at a time. You can use a Q-tip or one of the blunt objects that frequently come with a nail-trimming kit. The idea is to free the end of the nail from the adjacent skin, preventing the burrowing under that causes the problem.

We tell our patients to try to place a wedge of gauze or a piece of cotton under the nail or even a piece of dental floss—anything to keep the end of the nail free. One technique describes lifting the nail with a piece of cotton and then applying skin glue to form a kind of cast. You can leave this in place until it falls off on its own. So whatever it takes and whatever you're comfortable doing. In the movie *Braveheart*, the mantra was "Free-dom!" Here, it's "Free the nail!" And you don't have to wear a kilt. The important fact is that more than 70 percent of toes will respond to this kind of conservative therapy, so try to do something.

But if it's too late for that, if your teenager's big toe is so swollen and red and painful that he can barely walk on it, it's time for something more.

This is going to require some effective local anesthesia at a doctor's office, usually in the form of a nerve block—injecting an anesthetic that deadens the nerves that run on the outside of each toe. There's no magical way of doing this, and it's going to hurt. But then it's done, and your child's not going to feel anything further.

### ✛ *What about using some numbing cream?*

The most frequently used numbing cream is called EMLA, but it doesn't work on toes. We have to block those nerves.

The next step is to take some sharp, straight scissors (or a similar instrument) and remove a wedge of the nail all the way back to the base. Once that's done, any infected material needs to be removed along with any "proud flesh." Proud flesh refers to part of the normal healing process—pink/red tissue composed of newly formed blood vessels—that has gotten out of control. It spills over the nail and has to be removed. Trimming it away works, and then we cauterize it with a silver nitrate stick. This leaves the area blackened, but the discoloration will wear off in a couple of days. Twice-daily antibiotic cream and a covering bandage will be needed for several days, and the toe will need to be kept clean and dry. Oral antibiotics might be needed, too, depending on the presence and extent of infection, and acetaminophen or ibuprofen will usually handle the pain. Once we've gone to all this trouble (and pain!), we want to be sure that the child is wearing the correct shoes, trimming their nails correctly, and letting you know of any early redness and swelling.

Sometimes this problem will come back, and when it does, it will frequently need an even more aggressive approach. The nail will need to be "wedged" again, but this time the base (where the nail grows from) will have to be destroyed, either with a laser treatment or a chemical (phenol). This will need to be done by an orthopedist or podiatrist.

While not a terrible experience, we all want to avoid a treatment like this. And it can be avoided. As we said earlier, ingrown toenails can be prevented. Just pay attention.

> *"There are three ways to do things around here:*
> *the right way, the wrong way,*
> *or the way that I do it."*
>
> Ace Rothstein, *Casino*

# 34

# Eating Disorders

### ✚ *What should I look for if I think my teenage daughter has an eating disorder?*

This is a critical question, and the fact that you're asking it is the first and most important step.

EMS 2 had just taken a 16-year-old girl to the cardiac room and transferred her to our stretcher. The paramedics had called in a report of "unresponsive with no pulse," and nothing had changed before their arrival.

There was a flurry of organized chaos surrounding her bed as our team worked to get the teenager stabilized. She was skinny to the point of being wasted, and I wondered if she had some form of cancer.

Her mother had followed the EMS team into the room, and I turned to her. "Does your daughter have some serious illness? Cancer or kidney failure? Any medical problems?"

The woman stiffened, and her eyes narrowed. "Cancer? Of course not! Kylie's been perfectly fine until...maybe the last couple of days. She just hasn't seemed herself."

"Heart rate is 52," one of the nurses told me. "I can't get a blood pressure."

My eyes studied the mother's face, trying to find some opening, some chink in this wall of denial. We would need to talk.

I spun around to her daughter. "Get lab down here and X-ray!"

Eating disorders are all too common, with their prevalence increasing every year. Now that number is a little more than 3 out of every 100 people. That might not sound like many, but the rate of appendicitis—something we all worry about—is only 1 out of 400. And while we used to think of these disorders as only a problem among teenagers or maybe young women in their early twenties, those affected are getting younger and younger—as early as six and seven years of age. That should scare all of us. Eating disorders include binge eating, rumination disorder, pica, night eating, purging, avoidant/restrictive food intake disorder, and the two most familiar, anorexia nervosa and bulimia. Of these two, anorexia is the more serious and the more deadly. (We'll talk more about anorexia and bulimia in the next chapter.)

> "When it comes to adolescent eating disorders, it is usually the parents' responsibility to seek help. The girl with the eating disorder is often the last to know she is ill."
>
> **AMY BAKER**

We're not sure where these illnesses come from or what triggers them. One common denominator appears to be an unnatural and unhealthy perception of self-image, which can be manifested as early as in the preschool years. Whatever the cause, it's multifactored and includes family dynamics as well as peer and social media interaction.

And it's real. Unrecognized and untreated, these disorders can lead to heart muscle atrophy, other serious cardiac problems, osteoporosis, growth disturbance, life-threatening electrolyte abnormalities, and suicide. The diagnosis can be difficult and delayed, mainly because of that *wall of denial* I mentioned. This can be encountered with the young people themselves or with their parents. However, we need to be aware of a few telltale signs, especially with bulimia.

For instance, the frequent self-induced vomiting associated with bulimia produces calluses on the backs of several fingers (from eliciting a gag reflex) as well as a wasting away of the enamel of the teeth from exposure to the acid contents of the stomach. And then there's the weight loss of anorexia nervosa. Parents just don't notice these changes until their children are way down the road. The effects of eating disorders are gradual and can be difficult to detect when a parent sees their son or daughter every day. That's another important point—*son or daughter*. With many of these disorders, contrary to common thought, the incidence in boys is the same as in girls, so parents just have to be aware.

Fortunately, one simple tool can at least raise some red flags. The SCOFF questionnaire, developed by John Morgan at Leeds Partnerships NHS Foundation Trust in England, is simple and accurate enough to be an initial screen. If you're concerned about the possibility that your child has an eating disorder, these are the questions you should ask your child—or you can answer them from your own observations.

- Do you make yourself **S**ick [vomit] because you feel uncomfortably full?
- Do you worry you have lost **C**ontrol over how much you eat?
- Have you recently lost more than **O**ne stone [14 pounds] in a three-month period?
- Do you believe yourself to be **F**at when others say you are too thin?
- Would you say that **F**ood dominates your life?[1]

Two or more positive answers is cause for concern and are frequently indicative of an eating disorder. If that's your child's score, or if you have *any* concern that your child has an eating disorder, get help now!

For Kylie, that help came too late. She died two days later in the ICU—her mother still in denial.

> *"Understanding is the first step to acceptance,*
> *and only with acceptance can there be recovery."*
>
> Albus Dumbledore, *Harry Potter and the Goblet of Fire*

# 35

# Anorexia and Bulimia

✚ *What's the difference between anorexia and bulimia?*
*And is that difference important?*

There *is* a difference. And it *is* important.

## Bulimia Nervosa

The word "bulimia" comes from the Greek word meaning "ravenous hunger," and "nervosa" obviously refers to the emotional/nervous part of this condition.

Bulimia is an eating disorder characterized by binge eating followed by an abnormal emotional response resulting in purging. We need to understand binge eating. This happens to be an actual eating disorder and is the most common one in the United States, affecting somewhere between 2 and 3 percent of all Americans. This was initially known as "the night eating disorder," probably because of stealthy trips to the refrigerator for ice cream. We know now that it occurs during all hours of the day and is marked by consuming an amount of food that is definitely much more than what most people would eat in a similar period of time under the same circumstances. The individual experiences a sense of lack of control over eating during the episode (feeling they cannot stop eating or control what or how much they're eating), eats more rapidly than normal, frequently eats alone, and will eat until uncomfortably full. To make the bulimia diagnosis, this needs to happen at least once a week for three months.

### ✛ What do you mean by "purging"?

Most of us think purging is an episode of self-induced vomiting. Frequently that's the case, but other efforts to "purge" oneself of the excessive food and to lose weight might be taking laxatives, taking someone's diuretics (fluid pills), fasting, taking over-the-counter stimulants, and even excessive exercising. Purging is what causes the damage. Common findings are low blood pressure, rapid heartbeat, dry skin, and problems with electrolytes, especially a low potassium or chloride. The blood chemistry changes stem from the excessive vomiting and can cause serious problems.

As mentioned in the previous chapter, another telltale physical marker of this disease is calluses or scars on the backs of fingers, the result of repeated trauma from the front teeth during self-induced vomiting.

Frequent vomiting can also lead to inflammation and bleeding from the esophagus, bleeding from the stomach, menstrual irregularities, and ultimately, infertility in young women. From the *nervosa* component, we see low self-esteem, depression, anxiety, an increased incidence of substance abuse, and a higher risk of suicide and self-harm. This is a serious problem, and it's a common one. The estimate is that 1 to 2 percent of us can be diagnosed with bulimia at any point in time, with the ratio of females to males as high as 9:1.

You might think bulimia would be easy to diagnose, but it's not. Most sufferers don't want to talk about it, and many parents don't want to address it. Compounding all of that is the fact that most patients with bulimia are of *normal* weight. This is different from the binge eating we talked about earlier, and from what we will learn about anorexia nervosa.

It's important to keep in mind that there is some overlap among all the eating disorders, so if you become a little confused and wonder how to keep them straight, don't feel alone. It can be difficult to make the correct diagnosis, but with a good history from parents and a focused and thorough exam, it can be done.

That "good history from parents" can sometimes be elusive. Family members and loved ones frequently have a sense that something's going on and yet are reluctant to mention it. They shouldn't be. Sometimes a life hangs in the balance.

So what are some of the things that should make our parental antennae stand on end? Here are some things to watch for:

- frequent self-weighing
- obsessive calorie counting
- ritualistic eating behaviors, such as cutting food into extremely small pieces
- binge-eating behavior
- frequent trips to the bathroom after a meal
- a preoccupation with body image and weight
- misuse of over-the-counter laxatives and stimulants
- characteristic physical changes, such as dental problems, dry skin, and calluses on the backs of fingers

Remember, individuals with bulimia nervosa are frequently of normal size and weight. Still, this is a serious and life-threatening eating disorder. Be aware, and don't be afraid to bring up the subject. There's help out there, and bulimia can be successfully treated and its adverse health effects reversed.

## Anorexia Nervosa

While the findings of bulimia nervosa can be subtle, those of anorexia nervosa are far from it. Of all the eating disorders, this is the deadliest. It literally results in starvation and all the medical complications associated with it. We've all seen pictures of extreme cases and maybe wondered how anorexia could ever be missed and allowed to progress to the point of this person being in such an emaciated condition. We might even have friends or loved ones who have purposefully lost weight to an excessive degree and continue to do so. While the effects might appear obvious to an outside observer or even to parents, the sufferers of anorexia usually have no insight into what's happening to their body. They just have a strong desire to be thin and an aversion to any body fat—sometimes to the point of death.

We've known about this disorder for hundreds of years, but the name "anorexia," which means "no appetite," is a misnomer. Individuals with this have not *lost* their appetite. They suppress it to lose weight and attain what they believe is a desirable body image. Here's what we need to be looking for overall:

- a persistent restriction of energy intake (food) that leads to an abnormally low body weight

- an intense fear of gaining weight or becoming fat or persistent behavior that prevents weight gain

- a distorted perception of body weight and shape

### ✛ What constitutes an abnormally low body weight?

Most experts utilize the BMI (body mass index), a simple calculation that can be found at www.CDC.gov/healthyweight/assessing/bmi/index.html. You only need to know your child's height and weight to use this tool. Here are some general categories of low body weight:

- Mild: a BMI of 17 to 18.5

- Moderate: a BMI of 16 to 16.99

- Severe: a BMI of 15 to 15.99

- Extreme: a BMI less than 15

An example would be that of a teenage girl who is five feet six inches tall and weighs 102 pounds. She would be in the moderate category. The same girl weighing less than 90 pounds would be in the extreme group. Why is this important? Remember, this is about *starvation*, so let's consider what starving does to our bodies.

When humans are starved, their bodies start to break down protein and fat in an effort to maintain critical energy levels and cellular activities. As a result, cells start to shrink, and we see atrophy of the heart, brain, liver, intestines, and muscle. The severity of this depends upon the length and magnitude of the starvation. (In Auschwitz, where prisoners were intentionally starved, receiving only 300 to 400 calories a day, the life expectancy was about three months.)

With the starvation of anorexia nervosa, it's not uncommon to see cardiovascular complications, such as a reduced cardiac muscle mass, scarring, and heart valve problems. Absence of menstrual periods and infertility are well documented, as is the early development of osteoporosis. If self-induced vomiting is part of the picture, we'll see the same GI complications we do with bulimia. And, importantly, starvation will ultimately affect our bone marrow, resulting in dangerous anemias, low white-cell counts that can lead to overwhelming infections, and low platelet counts, causing easy bruising and uncontrolled bleeding.

This is all bad stuff, but does it go away with treatment? Sometimes, but not always. Changes in both the gray and white matter in the brain as well as those cardiac changes can last a lifetime. That's why we need to pay attention to signs and intervene as quickly as we can.

So what are we looking for in more detail? Here are some tips:

- Some skin changes should raise a red flag. Yellowing of the skin is commonly seen, as is dryness and scaling.

- Hair loss occurs, as well as evidence of the easy bruising noted above.

- Darkening of the skin can also be seen, as well as persistent itching.

- Slowly healing wounds can be a problem because of poor nutrition and an impairment of the immune/healing process.

- Something called "lanugo" should always make us suspicious. This is the development of fine, dark, downy hair on the trunk and face. We're not sure why or how this happens, but in the setting of unexplained weight loss, this is an important warning sign.

In addition to these physical findings, we need to be aware of these behavioral and psychological warnings, some of which we've already indicated:

- restlessness or hyperactivity
- a relentless and unfounded pursuit of thinness
- concerns about eating in public
- a fear of certain foods
- inhibited expression of emotions
- poor sleep
- a need to control one's environment
- inflexible thinking
- a lack of insight into the existence of a potential eating problem
- anxiety or depression
- an intentional resistance to treatment and weight gain
- an obsessive preoccupation with food manifested in unusual ways, such as hoarding food or collecting recipes
- constantly counting calories
- consistently overestimating the number of calories in food
- overusing condiments and artificial sweeteners
- food-related rituals, including cutting food into small pieces, avoiding certain colors of food, and keeping food separated on the dinner plate

We all could check off some of these behaviors, and occurring by themselves, they're not necessarily pathologic. But if consistent, worsening, and combined with the kind of weight loss we've considered, they point to a more significant problem. Again, anorexia is the most dangerous of the eating disorders, and if you think your child might be affected, get help.

Where can you turn? Your pediatrician or family physician is a good place to start. Another valuable source of accurate and helpful information is NEDA, the National Eating Disorders Association (www.natio naleatingdisorders.org). If you have any suspicion that your child could be suffering from an eating disorder, the most important thing is to *act*. It won't go away on its own, and at some point, it can become too late to do anything about it.

> *"Girls developed eating disorders when our culture*
> *developed a standard of beauty*
> *that they couldn't obtain by being healthy.*
> *When unnatural thinness became attractive,*
> *girls did unnatural things to be thin."*
>
> Mary Pipher

# 36

# The Strange Things We Eat

✦ *My teenage boy chews ice all day long—just like his father does. Is that okay, or should I do something about him?*

Do something about whom? Your husband or your son? If you're referring to your husband, good luck. If it's your son, you should be aware of a couple of things.

First, there's a well-defined condition called "pica"—the eating of non-nutritional substances such as paper, cloth, soap, starch, ash, dirt, metal, string, and, yes, ice. Its cause is unknown, and the diagnosis requires at least a month of such activity. It's not very appetizing, but it happens. We've seen a dozen or so cases over the years involving young children of eight years of age up to a pregnant 20-year-old.

The eight-year-old boy was sent to the ER by his family doctor with a diagnosis of appendicitis. The child had been vomiting for a day or so and had severe abdominal pain. But he didn't have a fever, and his exam didn't show signs of appendicitis. His mother was more worried about his constipation. A simple X-ray of his abdomen revealed the problem. Long strands of something were blocking most of his large intestine. It turned out to be his grandmother's knitting yarn, and by the time we were finished with him, we had enough yarn for a sweater.

The 20-year-old pregnant young lady came to the ER one day complaining of weakness and "sleeping a lot." She had a dangerously low blood pressure and was pale and clammy. Simple blood work uncovered a profound anemia, so low that a blood transfusion was in order. Our battle-tested charge nurse noticed something in the woman's large purse—an opened and half-empty box of Argo starch. Her mother explained that the starch was all the young woman wanted to eat, and she was eating about three boxes a day. While the starch itself didn't cause the anemia, the exclusion in her diet of any meaningful nutrition did.

That was a close call. Fortunately, most children with pica don't present in such an extreme condition. The parents have noted some odd eating behaviors and what they describe as a fixation on some of the above-noted substances. While not necessarily posing a life-threatening risk to the child, this is something to pay attention to. Frequently, this condition can be associated with anxiety, mental health disorders, and occasionally a place on the autism spectrum. A good physical and psychological/developmental exam is in order.

Now, about the ice eating...A little ice crunching never hurt anybody, though it may drive your significant other up the wall. On the other hand, *excessive* ice chewing can be entirely different, and it has its own name—pagophagia. Once again, the time frame here is at least a month of chewing and consuming an abnormal amount of ice. That amount hasn't been accurately clarified; it's just abnormal. The risks are much the same as with other types of pica, the main one being anemia, secondary to the absence of needed and nutritious food in the diet. It can also be associated with stress, anxiety, and obsessive-compulsive disorder. And of course, the constant crunching on ice can damage tooth enamel, leading to the cracking and chipping of teeth.

> "The chains of habit are too weak to be felt until they are too strong to be broken."
> **SAMUEL JOHNSON**

So if your teenager is chewing ice every day, or you catch him eating some peculiar substance frequently, don't brush it off. It might be a passing preoccupation, but it could be something that needs to be addressed. And while you might get away with constantly nagging at your husband to stop chewing ice, not so with your child. Easy does it here. Start with an open, calm, non-accusatory dialogue. And get some help.

*"Nothing so needs reforming as other people's habits."*

Mark Twain

# 37

# Circumcision

*We're expecting a boy in a couple of weeks—our first child. I was circumcised when I was a baby, and I want him to be circumcised too. My wife's not sure. Her sister says it's barbaric. What should we do?*

Deciding whether to have your son circumcised requires considering several important factors (and whether your sister-in-law is right or wrong). The preferences you—the parents—have are significant, and they're often influenced by the father's own circumcision status. Then there are the opinions of other family members and even friends, plus a desire for conformity and to fit in—or maybe more importantly, to not stand out. And, of course, centuries of religious tradition. Sorting out all of these factors is *your* work. *Our* job is to pre-sent you with the current medical facts—for and against— and to help you assess the risks and benefits for your son.

Before we do that, it might be interesting for you to know what other people are doing. The United States is the only country in the developed world where the majority of male infants are circumcised for nonreligious reasons. An estimate of the overall prevalence (for religious and nonreligious reasons) is somewhere around 80 percent of US males. This is least common in our Western states (only about 30 percent) and most common in the Midwest (more than 75 percent). The South and Northeast fall somewhere in between. The great

> "Just because something is traditional is no reason to do it, of course."
>
> **LEMONY SNICKET**

majority of these procedures are done with newborns, but a substantial number are performed on older children, teenagers, and even young adults. As many as 1 in 5 of those not circumcised at birth will elect to have it done later. These are the guys who walk funny for a couple of days and wish they had had the procedure when they were a few days old.

The benefits of circumcision are important and well established. Significantly, urinary tract infections (UTIs) are reduced by as much as 90 percent. That's a big number, and this is the major medical benefit during infancy. UTIs are uncommon in males at any age, but they are more prevalent in infants, when it can lead to life-threatening complications. This reduction in UTIs extends beyond infancy and throughout a man's entire life.

Circumcision has also been found to reduce the risk of some forms of cancer. For instance, circumcision produces a reduction in the incidence of penile cancer. This is a rare cancer (estimated to be less than 1 in 100,000 males), but studies demonstrate that circumcision provides a protective effect. Cervical cancer is more common in the sexual partners of uncircumcised men. The reason might be that uncircumcised men have a higher incidence of human papillomavirus (HPV), but with the widespread use of the HPV vaccine in women and men, this may become less of a factor.

Easier cleansing and improved hygiene leads to a reduction in the inflammatory problems more common in uncircumcised males. These include infections of the foreskin and glans itself, sometimes leading to scarring and the need for corrective surgery. While we're talking about cleaning, we need to say it's important to know how to properly clean your infant's penis. The foreskin needs to be completely retracted and the glans gently cleaned with soap and water. Look carefully for the presence of a hair encircling the glans; it can be hard to see. The two of us have observed multiple instances of this happening, usually when anxious parents bring their child to the office or ER with "something wrong with his *parts*." The hair can act as a tourniquet, causing swelling and infection. In the extreme, it can cut off blood flood to the glans and result in amputation. Not good.

Interestingly, circumcision has been proven to protect against the spread of HIV and herpes simplex virus type 2. Maybe even trichomonas, but not gonorrhea, chlamydia, or syphilis. The evidence for HIV is such that the World Health Organization (WHO) has recommended that male circumcision be a part of an HIV preventive plan in areas of the world where the infection is common.

✦ **What about the pain? I've read that my newborn will experience a lot of pain and that it might interfere with his breastfeeding. I also read that when he's older, he'll have less sensitivity and less, you know, satisfaction.**

Let's look at one question at a time. Yes, there are some complications associated with this procedure, but the risk is less than 0.2 percent (2 in 1,000). These include:

- *Bleeding.* This is usually mild and controlled with local pressure. Rarely, it can be severe and require surgical treatment.

- *Infection.* If the person doing the procedure is experienced and uses a sterile technique, this shouldn't happen. If it does, the infection is usually mild and needs only a topical antibiotic.

- *Inadequate skin removal.* This shouldn't happen with an experienced provider, but it can lead to a poor cosmetic appearance, resulting in a corrective operation at some point in the future.

- *Removal of too much skin.* Again, this is mainly a cosmetic problem.

- *Scarring and adhesions.* These are rare, but when significant, they might lead to another procedure.

All of these complications are more common among premature newborns, those with congenital anomalies, those whose circumcision is performed *after* the newborn period, and those whose circumcisions are performed by poorly trained providers. In a large teaching hospital, a first-year resident with little experience will sometimes be relegated to this task. Ask your obstetrician who's going to perform your baby's circumcision, what their level of experience is, and maybe even ask to meet them. Don't assume anything. This is a simple and safe procedure, but it has lifelong consequences.

About your pain question. This is a surgical procedure, and some degree of pain will be a reality. The good news is that the pain can be safely controlled with a couple of local anesthetic options. Not too long ago, this wasn't considered to be of great importance, but now every infant should be afforded relief of the anticipated discomfort. This is another question to ask the person who's going to do the procedure. Insist on that pain relief.

Regarding your concern about breastfeeding, with adequate pain management this should not be a problem. Any behavioral changes noted in your newborn, if any, shouldn't last more than 24 hours. And concerning your sensitivity issue, there is no evidence in the medical literature to expect this to be a problem.

On balance, most experts agree that the medical benefits of circumcision outweigh the risks. The American Academy of Pediatrics has developed a policy statement on this issue. We've included it here because we believe it presents an accurate and objective presentation of the current data and provides solid guidance for soon-to-be parents of male children.

> Systematic evaluation of English-language peer-reviewed literature from 1995 through 2010 indicates that preventive health benefits of elective circumcision of male newborns outweigh the risks of the procedure. Benefits include significant reduction in the risk of urinary tract infection in the first year of life and, subsequently, in the risk of heterosexual acquisition of HIV and the transmission of other sexually transmitted infections.

> The procedure is well tolerated when performed by trained professionals under sterile conditions with appropriate

pain management. Complications are infrequent; most are minor, and severe complications are rare. Male circumcision performed during the newborn period has considerably lower complication rates than when performed later in life.

Although health benefits are not great enough to recommend routine circumcision for all male newborns, the benefits of circumcision are sufficient to justify access to this procedure for families choosing it and to warrant third-party payment for circumcision of male newborns. It is important that clinicians routinely inform parents of the health benefits and risks of male newborn circumcision in an unbiased and accurate manner.

Parents ultimately should decide whether circumcision is in the best interests of their male child. They will need to weigh medical information in the contest of their own religious, ethical, and cultural beliefs and practices. The medical benefits alone may not outweigh these other considerations for individual families...

The American College of Obstetricians and Gynecologists has endorsed this statement.[1]

In the end, it's all about making a thoughtful and informed decision. This information informs you, and now you can give it some thought.

*"Whatever course you decide upon,*
*there is always someone to tell you that you are wrong.*
*There are always difficulties arising which tempt you*
*to believe that your critics are right.*
*To map out a course of action and follow*
*it to an end requires courage."*

Ralph Waldo Emerson

38

# Sorting Out
# Medical Literature

✚ *With everything out there on the internet,
whom are we to believe?*

The latest medical studies..."
"New research has shown..."
"My friend just told me..."

We hear it all the time. Some new medical claim is released, and the media floods the airways and internet with wild predictions based on this "latest and greatest" breakthrough. In moments, the claim becomes an established fact and the latest talking point. Then, as quickly as it appeared, it's gone. Not always, but that seems to be the rule rather than the exception.

Or you're trying to learn something about the signs and symptoms of diabetes, or your child has a bad sunburn and you want to know the best thing to do so you google "sunburn," and all kinds of tidbits pop up. And then ads start coming from every direction, and you don't know where to turn. Where do we find accurate, safe, and proven information?

How are we to deal with these life-changing discoveries? What are we to make of these claims and wild predictions? How do we sort out what's true from what's bluster and bling?

For the most part, our advice is to take these astonishing claims with a grain of salt.

## ✛ But, Doctors, you refer to "medical studies" and "recent research" in this book. How do you know what's factual and what's not?

That's the question, isn't it? And you're right, we do rely on numerous studies and articles as we present information on the various topics in this book. But we do so cautiously, keeping in mind that we want to give information that is accurate as well as up-to-date. We know a lot of bogus stuff is out there, and many medical studies are easily influenced by forces that are powerful and difficult to combat—usually in the form of money and usually with the backing of the pharmaceutical industry. We have to be careful when we look at any new study, especially when some new drug, treatment, or device is touted as "changing everything." Who's paying for the study, and are the researchers potentially influenced by them?

> "Get your facts first, then you can distort them as you please."
>
> **MARK TWAIN**

There's a lot to keep in mind here, and we don't have enough watchdogs looking out for us. But as a rule, if something sounds too good to be true, it probably is. And there's always the media, frequently guilty of overhyping medical claims that come across their desks. It doesn't matter that no supporting facts exist, only mainly conjecture or anecdote. But it doesn't take much to set off widespread confusion and even hysteria (cell phones causing cancer, aspartame causing a host of medical problems, anthrax on your doorstep).

Where do *we* turn for information? And how would we advise our readers to evaluate a new medical claim or look up some information about a particular illness, symptom, or treatment? First, we advise against blind surfing on the internet. You never know what you'll find—or where you'll end up. Usually it's in confusion, wild claims, and the opportunity to buy something that supposedly will change your life.

However, we can recommend a few websites with confidence. These are well-established and authoritative, and they cover many areas of medical care and recent research. These are places we go to answer questions that arise or to gain perspective on the latest medical miracle.

- www.CDC.gov—This is the CDC website, and we've referred to it on several occasions. This site has no-nonsense information, and information about everything. If something is out there in the community, you'll find help here.

- www.medlineplus.gov—This is a user-friendly site with a lot of good information.

- www.mayoclinic.org—This is another reputable and user-friendly site, and it's easy to navigate.

- www.health.harvard.edu—Hey, this is the Ivy League, right? They must know what they're talking about, and they do.

- my.clevelandclinic.org/health/default.aspx—The Cleveland Clinic is a highly regarded institution, and we've found their website to be current and useful.

- www.AAP.org—This is the website for the American Academy of Pediatrics, and you'll find it to be a complete and useful resource.

These should be enough websites to help you find whatever you're looking for. Check them out to see which ones you like. Just remember, when you hear some new claim of a miracle breakthrough or someone spouting "overwhelming evidence" in some new study, it's always wise to let the dust settle. Time has a way of dealing with most things, and the truth finds a way to declare itself. So be cautious—maybe even cynical—and keep in mind what Winston Churchill had to say on this topic. Unfortunately, he was right.

*"A lie gets halfway around the world
before the truth has a chance to put its pants on."*

Winston Churchill

# 39

# Fractured Medical Terms

*✚ My teenager is having palpations. What should we do?*

Do you mean "palpitations"? There's a difference between palpations and palpitations, and this might be a good time to focus on the use—and misuse—of medical terminology. Granted, a lot of the medical profession's language is derived from ancient Latin (almost all anatomical names), Greek (arthritis, nephritis, phobias), French (lavage, hemorrhage), and Old English (dropsy, palsy), and granted, many in our profession sometimes confuse and distort our own words. But it's still important to be able to communicate with each other. This is especially important when we're talking about health-related issues, so we need to at least come close to the proper word or phrase.

The following are examples of coming close, taken from the questionnaires and written forms of actual patients or from their verbal histories. (See if you catch the draft. Some are quite traffic.)

- scrip throat—strep throat
- rotor cup—rotator cuff
- technical shot—tetanus shot
- depositories—suppositories
- cadillac—cataract
- diarear—diarrhea
- buttocks—Botox
- acid reflex—reflux

- amtracks—anthrax
- herbal bowel syndrome—irritable bowel syndrome
- my brain headache—migraine
- prostrate/prospate—prostate
- Oltimer's disease—Alzheimer's disease
- Canada infection—candida (yeast) infection
- choirpracter—chiropractor
- gouch—gout
- sonotic nerve—sciatic
- smoking sensation classes—smoking cessation classes
- Tyrenol—Tylenol
- chicken pops—chicken pox
- smilin' mighty Jesus—spinal meningitis
- vomick/cascade—vomit
- fireballs in my Eucharist—fibroids of the uterus
- delighted—dilated
- aerial fiburation—atrial fibrillation
- Hi herny—hiatal hernia

And then there are the terms that make you want to scratch your head.

- artery—the study of painting
- seizure—one of the Roman emperors
- labor pain—getting hurt at work
- bacteria—the back door of a cafeteria
- outpatient—a person who has fainted
- PAP smear—a paternity test
- colic—a sheep dog

- tumor—more than one
- urine—opposite of you're out
- fester—someone who is quicker
- enema—not a friend
- Caesarean section—a neighborhood in Rome
- barium—what doctors do when a patient dies
- cat scan—search for a kitty
- node—was aware of
- vein—conceited
- terminal illness—getting sick at the airport
- hangnail—a coat hook
- dilate—to live long
- recovery room—a place to do upholstery
- varicose—nearby
- pelvis—a cousin of Elvis
- postoperative—a letter carrier
- nitrates—cheaper than day rates
- tablet—a small table
- impotent—distinguished, well known
- rectum—dang near killed 'em

As you can see, we sometimes need a translator. Fortunately, if we pay attention, we can decipher the intended meaning of a word or phrase. Taking Latin in high school was a big help in understanding the origin of medical words and how to use them. For those of us who didn't, learning medical terminology wasn't easy, and most of us needed some help. One popular and effective teacher of anatomy, understanding the limitations of the medical students sitting before him, broke down the essential anatomic structures of the chest cavity by describing the "birds of the thoracic cage."

- the esophagoose
- the thoracic duck (duct)
- the azygoose vein (azygos)
- the hemi-azygoose vein (a close cousin)
- the accessary hemi-azygoose vein (a distant cousin)
- the vagoose nerve (vagus)
- the peri-cardinal sac (pericardial)
- and the swallow—a stretch, but it still works

If that dispels a little of the mystery surrounding medical terminology and the process of medical education...well, good. Now what was that question about palpations?

*"Here will be an old abusing of God's*
*patience and the king's English."*

William Shakespeare

# 40

# Questions and Answers

Now it's our time to ask *you* some questions. Grab a pencil (make sure it has an eraser), and let's see how you do.

1. Your two-year-old has a temperature of 102.2. You've read that an ice pack, along with acetaminophen, will help bring it down. All you have is a bag of frozen peas. Where's the best place to put it?

   a. on your child's head

   b. on her exposed belly

   c. over both her thighs (but you'll need two bags of peas)

   d. back in the freezer

Easy, right? Put those peas back in the freezer. Not only will placing that bag on your child make her uncomfortable, but it's not going to help. Sponging with tepid water is the most extreme external treatment we recommend, but even that's not going to help much.

2. Which of the following, when swallowed by your three-year-old, will be safely passed through his GI system?

   a. one thin dime

   b. a paper clip

   c. a pushpin from a corkboard

   d. a medium-sized fishhook

   e. all of the above

The answer is all of the above. Each of these items has been documented as making it into a child's mouth and out the other end. The
critical point is the esophagus. If a foreign body makes it into the stomach, it should continue on through—although some things need to
be removed no matter where they are, like button batteries (they can
corrode and release dangerous chemicals) and two or more magnets,
even if they're small. The magnets can attach to each other, with a loop
of bowel in between. Over a short amount of time, this pressure and
rubbing together can perforate the bowel wall, causing infection and
major complications.

Yet, again, the GI tract is capable of safely passing many things,
some of which might seem impossible. Here's a list of items that have
been ingested and safely passed (not by the same person):

| | | |
|---|---|---|
| a spoon | an unopened safety pin | an opened safety pin |
| a straight pin | a ballpoint pen | assorted coins |
| a key | nails | a sharpened pencil |
| a small harmonica | a soft-drink cap | pieces of broken glass |
| a whistle | a small aspirin bottle | a wristwatch |
| checkers pieces | chess pieces | Monopoly pieces |
| tacks | pushpins | dice |
| a razor blade | a closed pocketknife | marbles |
| fishhooks | fish bones | fishing sinkers |
| ham bone | pork chop bones | toy soldiers |
| Legos | Lincoln logs | fuses |
| broken thermometers | teeth | false teeth |
| buttons | washers (not a Maytag) | bolts and screws |

Impressive, isn't it? And to think, back in the day we used to get into
big trouble if we swallowed our chewing gum.

3. Which of the following is true concerning conjunctivitis (pink eye)?

   a. It's very contagious.

   b. It's easy to distinguish between an allergic problem (seasonal allergies) or a bacterial infection.

   c. It can be spread simply by looking at someone.

   d. If bacterial, it almost always responds to warm compresses.

The only correct answer is *a*. Conjunctivitis, whether viral or bacterial, is extremely contagious. Seasonal allergies can be hard to distinguish from an infection. Both cause redness and usually some drainage. A couple of tips can help. The drainage from an allergic problem is usually clear, while the drainage from an infection is frequently yellow and sticky. Some experts tell us that if a child wakes up with her eyelids stuck together, that's a good indication of a bacterial infection. Another tip is that allergies almost always affect both eyes while an infection starts in only one. Warm compresses can help with the discomfort of conjunctivitis and help clean the eye, but with a bacterial infection, antibiotic drops are usually required to clear the problem.

4. Which of the following childhood diseases is considered benign?

   a. measles

   b. mumps

   c. H. flu infections (meningitis)

   d. whooping cough

   e. none of the above

None of these diseases are benign. Measles can cause serious complications, including death. Whooping cough is dangerous in the "extremes" of life—for those who are very young and those who are older than 75 or so. H. flu has caused many cases of meningitis with its predictable complications, but since the advent of an effective vaccine, this has become a rare occurrence. If you thought mumps wasn't a serious infection, think again. While we don't see many cases—thanks to the MMR—mumps can cause swelling and inflammation of the testicles and ovaries, an infection of the brain, and pancreatitis.

5. Which of the following is the most painful vaccine?

    a. Diphtheria-tetanus-pertussis

    b. H. flu

    c. MMR

    d. PCV (pneumonia)

While it's difficult to know for sure because young children aren't able to verbally communicate their level of pain, researchers have studied various responses and determined that this list of vaccines starts with the least painful and ends with the most painful. Some recommendations suggest starting with the least painful vaccine first. Here are also a couple of tips for reducing the anticipated pain your child will have with his scheduled shots.

- If he's breastfeeding, this should be done during the immunization process.

- A teaspoon of sugar dissolved in 10 cc's of water can be administered orally one to two minutes before the injection. (This works best in children less than 12 months of age.)

- A topical anesthetic cream will help, but it needs to be applied 30 to 40 minutes before the shot.

- A rapid technique of injection, rather than a slow one, is associated with less pain.

6. Which of the following is considered to be the "silent killer"?

    a. pinworms

    b. a broken heart

    c. too much cabbage and beans

    d. hypertension

If you answered *c*, then you probably don't have too many close friends. Pinworms might drive you to distraction, but they're not a killer. And a broken heart, while painful, can be mended. Hypertension is the silent killer. It hammers away at our brains and hearts and kidneys, and it can start at a young age. Your child should have yearly blood pressure checks, starting at three years of age. Fortunately, hypertension is uncommon when we're that young, but its incidence increases with each passing year. An elevated cholesterol is a risk factor for heart disease, and we need to check that level at 11 years of age. Know your numbers *and* your child's.

7. Which of the following causes the most common food allergy?

    a. cow's milk

    b. nuts

    c. eggs

    d. soy products

    e. shrimp

While all of these foods can cause food allergies, the most common offender is anything in the nut family. These allergies can present at any time, but usually after the age of one. Most experts suggest introducing known potential allergens from six months to one year because this can help a child develop tolerance and forestall a full-blown allergy. That strategy doesn't always prevent it, but it can help. If you try this, make sure your pediatrician is on board and that you introduce one such food item at a time. Frequently encountered symptoms include cough, swollen lips, and welts. Wheezing and shortness of breath are unusual findings. Milk protein allergies can present with violent vomiting and bloody stools.

8. Which of the following is or are true concerning birth-order characteristics?

   a. Firstborn children tend to be organized and rule followers. They have narrow mood swings, never being super happy or super sad. They're reluctant to try new things because of the fear of failure and tend to be introverted. They usually do well in school and will have only a few good friends, maybe just one.

   b. Middle children are strong-willed and risk takers. They have wider mood swings and are fearless and messy. They're your rule breakers.

   c. Last children are a good combination of *a* and *b*. Flexible and funny, they're the family entertainer. They're extroverted and have many friends.

   d. All of the above (and usually the firstborn child will be the oldest)

The answer is *d*. If you have several siblings, see if this breakdown rings true. This is interesting stuff, and it can help you understand your children a little better and help explain some of their behaviors. Maybe even your own.

9. What's the best treatment for a helicopter mom and an aerial-drone dad?

   a. Tie their hands behind their back.

   b. Make them wear shock collars.

   c. Take away their car keys and cell phones.

d. Do whatever else it takes.

e. All of the above

Again, the answer is all of the above. Being a helicopter mom or aerial-drone dad will wear you out and strain every family relationship. And rather than helping your children, it will hinder their development of effective coping skills. In addition, the constant hovering can increase their level of anxiety and ultimately lead to depression.

10. Is it "starve a fever and feed a cold" or "feed a fever and starve a cold"?

   a. Both are correct.

   b. Both are wrong. It should be "give everyone chicken soup."

   c. Both are goofy.

   d. You're talking about an inaccurate old wives' tale, so forget about it.

The answer is *d*. You don't have to worry about keeping this fourteenth-century medical axiom straight. It doesn't matter because both are inaccurate. Whether we have a cold or a fever, we need adequate and balanced nutrition in addition to plenty of fluids. Chicken soup might be good for the soul, but it's loaded with salt and might worsen any condition that causes fluid loss and potential dehydration.

11. Children will usually outgrow which of the following:

   a. asthma

   b. ear infections

   c. febrile seizures

   d. blue eyes

   e. all of the above

Did you choose all of the above? If you did, good for you. Childhood asthma improves over time, frequently because the wheezing we hear and treat is not classic asthma but some other type of allergic problem. Ear infections decrease in frequency after a child reaches three or four years of age. This is because of the changing anatomy of the Eustachian tube as the head and neck areas mature. Febrile seizures can recur for a couple of years, but age five seems to be the time when most stop. And blue eyes are common in newborns, only to change in color over the next few weeks and months.

12. Which of the following are symptoms of depression?

> a. lack of energy
>
> b. problems with sleeping
>
> c. feelings of sadness
>
> d. loss of interest in the things that previously gave joy
>
> e. difficulty concentrating
>
> f. changes in appetite resulting in weight loss or weight gain
>
> g. all of the above

The incidence of depression is steadily increasing among our adolescents, and all of these are frequently experienced symptoms. It's estimated that at any one point in time, 8 percent of our teenagers have some degree of depression. All too often this goes unrecognized and untreated. When that happens, the risk of suicide increases. That's now the second leading cause of death of those 5 to 24 years of age. This is happening in every part of our country, in every neighborhood, and to kids from all walks of life. Here's what it looks like.

> A 15-year-old girl takes an overdose of her mother's pain pills. She's upset with her boyfriend and "doesn't want to live anymore." She survives this attempt, is seen by a

psychiatrist, and seems to be doing better. Two months later she tries again, and this time she succeeds.

A 16-year-old boy is upset with his parents and is having trouble in school. He takes the shotgun his grandfather gave him into the backyard, places the barrel against his chest, and pulls the trigger.

A 19-year-old college freshman becomes depressed during her second semester. She writes a good-bye note, leaves it on the bed in her dorm, gets into her car, and drives into a concrete column of an interstate overpass going 90 miles an hour.

It's happening, and we'd better pay attention.

13. When it comes to lacerations, which of the following are true statements?

   a. Dermabond (skin glue) can be used on any laceration up to one inch in length.
   b. Redness of a half inch surrounding the wound is a sign of infection.
   c. Staples in the face, if they're small, are safe to close a laceration.
   d. Once healed, the scar will be stronger than the original skin.
   e. None of the above.

None of these are true. Skin glue, when used properly, can give an excellent cosmetic result. The length of the laceration is not as important as the *tension* across it. If the wound is gaping, skin glue shouldn't be used. Nonetheless, many parents want the glue because the process doesn't involve a needle stick, pain, or screaming. But it's the cosmetic result we're concerned with.

The normal healing process includes an *inflammatory* process that brings in the cells necessary for crucial functions. This will cause redness, which doesn't mean infection.

Staples should never be used on the face, no matter how small they are. If your physician reaches for a staple gun, reach for the door.

A healed wound/scar will never be as strong as it was before—maybe only 75 percent.

14. Which of the following is true regarding a CT scan of your child's abdomen?

    a. It has the same radiation exposure as 400 chest X-rays.

    b. It will increase the risk of your child developing a fatal cancer.

    c. It has a little more radiation than an ultrasound.

    d. It has the same radiation as an MRI.

*A* is correct, which is a lot, and that's what makes *b* correct as well. Depending on the area of the body scanned, we will see increases in the incidence of leukemia and brain tumors. But we need to keep a couple of things in mind. Each of us has a 1 in 5 chance of developing a fatal cancer during our lifetimes without any radiation exposure. The risk of one CT scan causing a fatal cancer is about 1 in 2,000. If we do a little math, without a CT our risk is 400 in 2,000 (1 in 5) and *with* a CT scan it becomes 401 in 2,000. That's not much of an increase, but it's definitely there.

The risk goes up with multiple scans. An ultrasound generates no radiation exposure, and in the right hands it's a good first choice for several conditions. An MRI is more expensive than a CT scan, but it doesn't expose you to any radiation. If your physician or an ER doctor is recommending a CT scan for your child, ask her if it's absolutely necessary. And then ask her if she would order one for her child.

15. What do we know about the "five second rule" (the law of nature that tells us we can safely eat an item of food that's been on the floor or ground for less than five seconds)?

a. This rule has been scientifically studied.

b. Bacteria and viruses require at least 14 seconds to attach to food.

c. A carpeted surface is much dirtier and more dangerous than a tiled floor.

d. The rule doesn't matter to a two-year-old because he's going to pick up whatever he dropped and put it in his mouth.

*A* and *d* are correct. For some reason, reputable people have studied this "rule" and come up with some interesting conclusions. Bacteria and other bugs can attach to dropped food in less than five seconds—sometimes immediately. Contrary to what we might think, carpet doesn't pose as much of a risk as does a clean-appearing tiled floor. And we all know about the two-year-old. Try to stop him.

The best advice is to forget the five second rule and forget what you or your child drops on the floor. However, the maternal grandfather of one of the authors was fond of saying that each of us will eat a "peck" of dirt in our lifetime. That's the equivalent of two dry gallons—a lot of dirt you don't want to eat at one sitting.

16. Match the following with the numbers 5, 2, 1, and 0.

a. hours of exercise your child needs each day

b. recommended number of daily servings of fruits and vegetables

c. allowable sugar drinks per 24 hours

d. hours of daily screen time for your child (TV, electronic devices, and so on)

Easy, right? The correct answers: a. 1; b. 5; c. 0; d. 2.

17. The following statements are true regarding potty training:

a. A more accurate term is "parent training."

    b. Don't consider starting before age 2.

    c. Positive reinforcement works best.

    d. Negative reinforcement and punishment should be avoided.

    e. Girls will be easier and quicker to train.

    f. All of the above.

All of these are correct—especially the one about parent training. Girls can successfully be trained by the age of three while boys will take longer. Three and a half to four years of age is considered normal.

Okay, did you get them all correct? If so, give us a call, and you can help write the next book!

# Closing Thoughts

Anne Denton was standing in the exam room, watching as her two-year-old son, Robert, played quietly with some Lego characters she'd brought from home. It was time for his scheduled well-child appointment, and she had noted "no specific concerns" on the intake form. Robert was walking and talking as he should according to everything she had read. He had always occupied the upper end of the growth chart for his height, and he was right in the middle for weight. And for the past six months he had been remarkably free of any of the coughs, colds, and crud that made the rounds among the children of their friends. He was their first child and doing great.

> "We may not be able to prepare the future for our children, but we can at least prepare our children for the future."
>
> **FRANKLIN D. ROOSEVELT**

Yet she had some lingering doubts. What about his diet? Was she feeding him the right things? And when should they begin the potty-training process? What about interaction with other children? Was he getting enough? And what about...

"Any other questions?" her pediatrician asked at the end of the visit.

There was a momentary silence as she looked down at her son. Then her eyes searched those of her doctor. "Do you think he's normal?"

There it was. *Is my child normal?* That's the question every concerned and involved parent asks. It comes from a deep place of love and commitment, tinged with anxiety and fear for the shadowy things of this world that await him—for those scary times when we won't be there to help. Whether or not Anne knows it yet, she's really asking,

199

"Will my child be all right? Will he be able to make it in this world on his own? Are we doing everything we can?"

We've spent the pages of this book providing guidance to help you with your child's health and safekeeping. That's a full-time job for a lot of years. But there's more to parenting than changing diapers, tending to countless bumps and bruises, and helping your children deal with complex medical problems. Much more. It's about preparing them for the journey ahead. That involves being a *good* parent, something that's intentional, sacrificial, and never-ending. But what does good parenting look like?

If we're fortunate, each of us has seen glimpses of good parenting as good parents have passed through our lives. Maybe they're still with us—family, friends, our own parents. For the two of us, the parents or caregivers of our patients have been models. They have demonstrated through their lives and actions what this guidance and sacrificial involvement encompasses.

First, there's a commitment of *time*. Hours, days, and years fly by, filled with the necessary but mundane activities of seeing that your child is fed, clothed, and protected. It's the *quality* time that all too often eludes us. Time taken out of our own busy lives, time devoted only to our children. One-on-one walks and talks, sharing thoughts and ideas, giving them the chance to share what's on their hearts—maybe what's on *our* heart. Those opportunities are slipping away.

Then there are our *words*. How do we speak to our children? Are the things we say building them up or tearing them down? This is where we need to step back and listen to ourselves speak. Our words, no matter how insignificant and unimportant we might think them to be, will have a profound and lasting impact on those little ears placed in our care. Anna Quindlen perceptively makes this point when she says, "Raising children is a spur-of-the-moment, seat-of-the-pants sort of deal, as any parent knows, particularly after an adult child says that his most searing memory consists of an offhand comment in the car on the way to second grade that the parent cannot even dimly recall."[1] Hmm...

Once spoken, our words can never be taken back, never be withdrawn. It's a constant struggle, guarding our tongues, words spoken in anger or impatience with lasting consequences. The thirteenth-century poet Rumi said, "Raise your words, not your voice. It is rain that grows flowers, not thunder." We need to make it our intention and our habit to use words that empower our children and communicate our love for them.

Sometimes we communicate our love *without* words. Our actions and the examples we give to our children speak loudly. That can be scary—or it can be an incredible opportunity. It's a choice. Our children are watching us and learning. A poem titled "When You Thought I Wasn't Looking" by Mary Rita Schilke Korzan beautifully makes this point.

> When you thought I wasn't looking
> You hung my first painting on the refrigerator
> And I wanted to paint another.
>
> When you thought I wasn't looking
> You fed a stray cat
> And I thought it was good to be kind to animals.
>
> When you thought I wasn't looking
> You baked a birthday cake just for me
> And I knew that little things were special things.
>
> When you thought I wasn't looking
> You said a prayer
> And I believed there was a God that I could always talk to.
>
> When you thought I wasn't looking
> You kissed me good-night
> And I felt loved.
>
> When you thought I wasn't looking
> I saw tears come from your eyes
> And I learned that sometimes things hurt—
> But that it's alright to cry.
>
> When you thought I wasn't looking
> You smiled
> And it made me want to look that pretty too.

When you thought I wasn't looking
You cared
And I wanted to be everything I could be.

When you thought I wasn't looking
I looked…and wanted to say thanks
For all those things you did
When you thought I wasn't looking.[2]

How we live, how we interact with our spouses and treat others—all of these things teach and inform our children. Being a parent isn't easy, is it?

Finally, we have *love*. This is what it's all about, isn't it? The fierce, enduring, and at times undefinable affection and devotion we have for our children. But as with all aspects of our lives, we're imperfect in love as well. Love requires sacrifice, a loss of self, a redirection of our hearts and minds—things that don't come naturally to us. Our minds need to be renewed and our hearts softened, and we need help doing it. We've been given examples of this—directions for what this looks like—through the life and teachings of Jesus.

The Lord speaks to us through the words of the apostle Paul when he tells us about love in his letter to the Corinthians. First Corinthians 13:13 says, "These three remain: faith, hope and love."

These words apply to all aspects of our lives, and we believe they guide us as parents. It's with *faith* that we take the leap to become parents in the first place. Faith that all will be well and that we are embarking on one of the greatest and most important journeys of our lives. *Hope* keeps our hearts and eyes focused on the future and on the promises we've been given. *Love* guides and assures us. It's the bedrock, the cornerstone of our relationship with our children. It endures.

> "Look for truth within yourself…Live a life of simplicity, love, and service. Let your life speak, and trust that your children will learn by your example."
>
> **ROBERT LAWRENCE SMITH**

The office visit was over. Anne Denton stopped at the front desk and made her son's next appointment. She held Robert's hand as they walked through the clinic doors, down the sidewalk, and into his future.

*"The greatest of these is love."*

1 Corinthians 13:13

# Index

# Notes

**Chapter 2. Helicopter Mom and Aerial-Drone Dads**

1. Malinda Carlson, "10 Warning Signs That You Might Be a Helicopter Parent (and How to Stop)," https://afineparent.com/be-positive/helicopter-parent.html.

**Chapter 3. Vaccinations**

1. Offit, Quarles, Gerber, et al., "Addressing parents' concerns: do multiple vaccines overwhelm or weaken the infant's immune system?" *Pediatrics* (2002):109, https://www.ncbi.nlm.nih.gov/pubmed/11773551.

**Chapter 4. Bullying**

1. James Rapp, Frank Carrington, and George Nicholson, *School Crime and Violence: Victims' Rights* (Pepperdine University Press, 1986, 1992), 18, https://www.ncjrs.gov/pdffiles1/Digitization/161362NCJRS.pdf.

**Chapter 7. Febrile Seizures**

1. Adapted from Offringa, Bossuyt, Lubsen, et al., "Risk factors for seizure recurrence in children with febrile seizures: a pooled analysis of individual patient data from five studies," *Journal of Pediatrics* (1994): 124:574, https://www.ncbi.nlm.nih.gov/pubmed/8151472.

**Chapter 8. Gastroenteritis and Dehydration**

1. David W. Kimberlin, MD, ed., *Red Book: 2018 Report of the Committee on Infectious Diseases, 31st Edition* (American Academy of Pediatrics, 2018), 577, 700, https://shop.aap.org/red-book-2018-paperback/.

**Chapter 9. Sleep**

1. Adapted from "Recommended Amount of Sleep for Pediatric Populations," *Journal of Pediatrics* (2016): 138; and Paruthi, D'Ambrosio, et al., "Recommended Amount of Sleep for Pediatric Populations: A Consensus Statement of the American Academy of Sleep Medicine," *Journal of Clinical Sleep Medicine* (2016) 12:785, https://aasm.org/resources/pdf/pediatricsleepduration-consensus.pdf.

2. Iglowstein, Jenni, Molinari, and Largo, "Sleep duration from infancy to adolescence: reference values and generational trends," *Journal of Pediatrics* (2003) 111:302, https://www.ncbi.nlm.nih.gov/pubmed/12563055.

3. Partuthi, D'Ambrosio, et al., "Recommended Amount of Sleep for Pediatric Populations: A Consensus Statement of the American Academy of Sleep Medicine," *Journal of Clinical Sleep Medicine* (2016) 12:785, https://aasm.org/resources/pdf/pediatricsleepdurationconsensus.pdf.

**Chapter 14. ADHD—Diagnosis**

1. Barkley, Cox, "A review of driving risks and impairments associated with attention-deficit/hyperactivity disorder and the effects of stimulant medication on driving performance," *Journal of Safety Research* (2007) 38:113, https://www.ncbi.nlm.nih.gov/pubmed/17303170.

2. American Psychiatric Association, "Attention-Deficit/Hyperactivity Disorder," *Diagnostic and Statistical Manual of Mental Disorders*, 5th Edition (American Psychiatric Association: Arlington, VA, 2013) 59.

3. Franke, B. et. al, "The Genetics of Attention Deficit/Hyperactivity in Adults, a Review," *Molecular Psychiatry*, October 2012, 17(10): 960-87.

**Chapter 22. SIDS**

1. Blair, Fleming, Smith, et al., "Babies sleeping with parents: a case-control study of factors influencing the risk of the sudden infant death syndrome," *British Medical Journal* (1999) 319:1457, https://www.ncbi.nlm.nih.gov/pubmed/10582925.

**Chapter 34. Eating Disorders**

1. "The SCOFF Questionairre," King's College London, https://www.leedsandyorkpft.nhs.uk/our services/wp-content/uploads/sites/2/2018/08/SCOFF-Questionnaire.pdf.

**Chapter 37. Circumcision**

1. American Academy of Pediatrics, "Circumcision Policy Statement," https://pediatrics.aappub lications.org/content/130/3/585.

**Closing Thoughts**

1. Anna Quindlen, *Living Out Loud* (New York, NY: Random House, 1988), 138.

2. Mary Rita Schilke Korzan, "When You Thought I Wasn't Looking," © 2004. Reprinted with permission of Andrews McMeel Publishing. All rights reserved.

# About the Authors

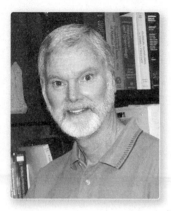

Bestselling author **Robert Lesslie** is a physician with more than 30 years experience in fast-paced, intense ER environments. He is now the co-owner and medical director of two urgent-care facilities. He has written many books, including *Angels in the ER* (over 200,000 copies sold), as well as newspaper and magazine columns and human-interest stories. He and his wife, Barbara, live in South Carolina.

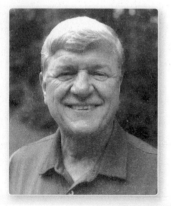

**Robert Alexander** has been a full-time practicing pediatrician since 1982 and has served as chief of the medical staff at Piedmont Medical Center in Rock Hill, South Carolina. He has also served on the Bioethics Committee of the South Carolina Medical Association and speaks regularly on the subject. Robert and his wife, Jeanie, have three adult sons and eight grandchildren.